Medicine of the Five Rings

Medicine of the Five Rings

和漢薬

How You Can Use New Japanese Herbal Medicines for Fitness, Vitality, and Health

Robert Rister

M. Evans and Company, Inc.
New York

DISCLAIMER:

This book provides information about the use of dietary supplements and other nonmedical healing practices as part of a broader program for the maintenence of general health. It is in no way intended to substitute for necessary medical diagnosis, advice, or treatment. This book is sold with the understanding that neither the publisher nor the author is liable for any damage resulting from the application or misapplication of any information presented in this book.

M. Evans and Company, Inc.
216 East 49th Street
New York, New York 10017

Library of Congress Cataloging-in-Publication Data

Rister, Robert
Medicine of the five rings : how you can use new Japanese herbal medicines for fitness, vitality, and health / Robert Rister
p. cm.
Includes bibliographical references and index.
ISBN 0-87131-977-2
1. Herbs—Therapeutic use—Japan. I. Title.
RM666.H33 R573 2002
615'.32'0952—dc21 2002067738

Typesetting and book design by Evan Johnston

Printed in the United States of America

9 8 7 6 5 4 3 2 1

Contents

Part 3. The Supplemental Medicines of the Five Rings

Acknowledgments

Kampo is a healing art learned under the forebearance of others. Many people have helped me learn this ancient method of herbal therapy, and several have been especially helpful in the preperation of this book.

Dr. Dan Wen, an individual of extraordinary intellectual presence, a teacher and researcher of both Western and Oriental medicine at some of the most prestigious institutions of both the People's Republic of China and the United States, and president of Honso USA, graciously and generously gave his time and support during the research of this book. Mr. Gyo Kinoshita, vice-president of Honso Pharmaceuticals in Japan also gave liberally of his time and knowledge in hosting me during my research in Osaka and Tokyo.

Several people offered helpful comments and criticisms in the writing of this book. Mr. Hideo Anzai of Tsumura USA and Dr. Andrew Vickers of Sloan-Kettering refined my understanding of some of the clinical applications of Kampo. Marcia Dean and Brian Johnson offered suggestions concerning style and language to make a complex subject readable. My editor Mark Gates verified cross-references for 84 traditional herbal remedies offered in over a dozen proprietary formulations and used in two medical systems for over 100 health conditions. And without the contributions of this book's designer, Evan Johnston, publication would not have been possible.

The true credit for any value of my presentation of this healing method, however, belongs to its founders and practitioners in Japan. The ingenuity and integrity of the sages of Kampo gave the world a unique form of natural medicine. The persistence and technical acumen of the modern manufacturers of Kampo have preserved this healing art for our time. Any demerit for failures of this presentation of this healing art is, of course, my own.

Preface

"You must research this well," admonished the Japanese master of martial arts Miyamoto Musashi. "This must be studied and practiced."

Like millions of other North Americans, my first exposure to the culture of Japan was through *The Book of Five Rings*. This bestseller was a translation of the sixteenth-century samurai's manual to the arts of war. Forced to wage battle against a samurai at the age of twelve, Musashi survived sixty battles by the age of sixty years, but lived to see Japan enter a time of peace.

As a *sensei*, a master teacher, Musashi recalled the essential elements of the samurai tradition in his book. He counseled the cultivation of a sense of timing, knowing the opponent, perseverance, and inner calm. Nearly four hundred years after its writing, his book remains a classic of Japanese literature.

Also like millions of other North Americans, I read the book but did not master any of the martial arts. I drifted from an aborted career in chemistry, to work with an international industrial efficiency consultant, to a failed attempt to become an herb farmer. That is, I drifted in my own professional purpose until, in 1984, I met my own *sensei*, an Austrian veterinarian named Helmut Bacowsky.

A practitioner of both veterinary and human medicine, who now directs a Kampo hospital for human patients in Europe, Dr. Bacowsky is an unlikely master of traditional Japanese Kampo medicine. When we met, he was also traveling through Asia. Helmut was taking a break from writing his dissertation on bone development in chickens for the School of Veterinary Medicine at the State University of Vienna. I was consulting on industrial efficiency to a maker of washing machines in the Philippines. Independently, we had both decided to take a weekend trip to the famed rice terraces around the village of Banaue, perched in the highlands of the Philippine island of Luzon.

That Sunday night a terrific rainstorm struck Banaue and washed out all the roads. Unfortunately, Helmut needed to get to Manila in two days to make a connection for a further trip to Australia, and I needed to depart to the United States before my visa expired the following Wednesday. We met while hiking over a mudslide to catch a jeepney to take us down the mountain to the nearest town.

Hanging on the railings outside the minibus—to allow room for pigs, chickens, and bags of fertilizer within—Helmut and I struck up a very long conversation on an exciting "new" method of health treatment he had learned with his wife in Japan. This was the system of herbal medicine the Japanese called the "China way" of treatment: Kampo. These precisely formulated herbal medicines were getting remarkable results in clinics in Japan, and he looked forward to returning to Austria—and to medical school, to get an M.D.—to use them.

Helmut Bacowsky became my *sensei*. He wrote the first textbook in English on Kampo medicine, and became a licensed physician. For ten years he sent me books and papers about Kampo in German, Japanese, and sometimes English. He discussed cases with me so that I might learn the craft. In time, I had the opportunity to round out my own learning experience with a research institute in Germany and began to publish books and articles about herbs in general and Kampo in particular. Under the crush of information available to me, I came to appreciate the kindness of my teacher Helmut Bacowsky and his wife, Michiko Okita. And, learning that Japanese herbal medicine began as an extension of the martial arts, I gained a new perspective on the writings of the Japanese master Musashi.

When the opportunity arose to write this book, I remembered the warning to research matters well. I attempted to read every available scientific article about laboratory and clinical tests of traditional Japanese herbal medicines. I located every book in English and the European languages on Japanese medicine, and some of the books in Japanese, and I made an effort to consult with every authority on the subject I could find in the United States. I also planned a research trip to Japan.

After months of delays, I finally had an appointment with one of Japan's practicing masters of herbal medicine. I brushed up key expressions in conversational Japanese and practiced my bow in front of a mirror. I put on my best dark suit. I made sure my business cards were in pristine condition. I was not quite over an especially stubborn case of bronchitis with inexplicable attacks of asthma, but I thought I could hold my cough for a few hours to get through the interview. The interview was not to go as I expected.

I arrived at the clinic and was escorted to the main office to see the master. I bowed. I was introduced as the apprentice of an Austrian *sensei* and a student of Kampo for 17 years. My host frowned in silence. His first question to me was, "How long have you been studying Kampo medicine?" "Since 1984," I answered. He then grimaced again and intoned, "You mean to say, for only 17 years?"

Sensing that the interview was already lost, I answered in the affirmative. "In that case," the master commented, "you have too little experience with herbal medicine for us to have a meaningful conversation. However, please stick out your tongue."

I complied, and this master of herbal treatment then held up a mirror. "Note," he said, "the white ridge in the center of your tongue and the red splotch on the front of your tongue. You have had bronchial asthma for three months." I in fact had had difficulty breathing for three months. "Moreover, you recently began to experience diarrhea, just a few days ago. It is due to the weakened condition of your lungs." I had suffered diarrhea in the week since I had arrived in Japan, and I knew it could not possibly be due to food contamination. I assumed my intestinal flora were simply unaccustomed to Japanese food.

The master then showed me a wheel divided into five parts. "These divisions," he said, impatiently reading their Japanese labels to me, "represent the Five Elements." "I assume my illness is due to . . ." I started. "Water," he finished. He then handed me an herbal powder with instructions to go to bed for three days. I recognized the formula as one designed to stimulate the kidneys, not the lungs, but I took it anyway—and after three days in bed I was recovered enough to resume my travels comfortably.

I was fortunate through the rest of my trip to meet a number of practical healers who treated patients with Kampo medicine on an everyday basis. Although the system of the Five Elements is more commonly associated with Chinese medicine, every practitioner I visited in Japan made use of the concept in making a swift diagnosis by looking at the patient and categorizing symptoms in terms of the Five Elements. And in Tokyo I met an acupuncturist, who, in the middle of a three-hour monologue on the use of lasers in making acupuncture needles, made an enlightening comment. "You realize, by the way," he said to me, "the Five Elements are just five kinds of coincidences. They are rings of circumstances that point to the causes and cures of every condition. To us, the concepts are second nature, but you will be able to use them to create a uniquely North American explanation of Kampo." He thereupon resumed his monologue on the modern machine tooling of acupuncture needles.

Maeda-san, the needle maker, had given me the insight I needed to write a new explanation of Kampo. The principles of Five Elements are well established in Chinese medicine. The idea that they correspond to "rings" of events inside and outside the human body is not a novel one; it is an extension of some of the ideas of Miyamoto Musashi. It is merely a new packaging of the basic principles of Japanese herbal medicine. It is, in part, a catalogue of symbols and interrelationships of the outside world and the health and disease processes inside the human body. And like any good analogy, the analogies of the Medicines of the Five Rings serve best when they are not pressed.

This book, of course, can never replace the practical wisdom dedicated healers acquire over decades of practice. Fortunately for writers, no system of herbal healing is more simplified or systematic than Japanese Kampo. It is versatile in that in can be understood in terms of yin, yang, the vital energy qi, and the Five Elements of Traditional Chinese Medicine, as it is in daily practice in Japan. It can also be understood in terms of the biology and pharmacology of the West, making it equally useful to devotees of energy healing as to scientifically trained health professionals. Therefore I have written this book in the hope that it can profit readers of Asian, Western, or eclectic orientation. In whatever way the formulas of Kampo medicine are understood, they work.

In the English-speaking world, Kampo medicine is an underutilized tool of natural healing. It is my sincere hope that you will find the herbal formulas described in this book to be of the highest quality and efficacy. I hope that you will find that the principles explained in this book speed you on your way to health.

How to Use This Book

If you are reading this book, chances are you already know the healing power of herbal medicine. You know that herbs are the most effective treatment of many common health conditions. They are free of side effects when chosen wisely. They are safe, natural, effective, and economical. The challenge for you is finding products of absolutely reliable quality. As you will read in this book, there are no herbal products of more reliable quality and no herbs that have been more thoroughly researched than the modern Japanese natural medicines known as Kampo.

This book presents eighty-four Kampo patent medicines that have recently become available across North America. These herbal formulas imported from Japan are already in use in every state of the United States and in every province of Canada. They are prescribed by naturopaths and enlightened physicians. They are available from herb shops, pharmacies, health-food stores, online health product sites, and supermarkets.

Kampo formulas are ancient herbal treatments. The manufacturers of Kampo products in Japan follow exactly the recipes written by the masters of Traditional Chinese Medicine as long as 1,700 years ago. Kampo formulas are energy medicines. That is, they are combinations of herbs designed to move the life force into its proper channels to restore balance and health, just as the masters of medicine prescribed them centuries ago.

Kampo formulas are also modern herbal treatments. Manufactured under exacting standards of sanitation and quality, these over-the-counter patent medicines provide familiar herbs of reliable quality. Because the content of Japanese herbal medicines is a known factor, it has been possible to begin to test Kampo formulas in Japan in the same manner that prescription drugs are tested in the United States. Every formula in this book has been tested at least in the laboratory and sometimes in controlled clinical studies. The principal components of every product described in this book are understood in terms of dosage, absorption, physiological effects, and interaction with prescription drugs.

Part 1 of this book offers an overview of the fundamental principles of Kampo as energy medicine. In the first chapter of Part 1, you will read about the unique historical influences that established a tradition of honest herbal medicine in Japan. In the second chapter you will read learn about the mysterious life force called *ki*. This is the energy that expresses itself as Yang and Yin. This fundamental concept underlies not only the East Asian traditions of herbal healing but also disciplines as diverse as feng shui and karate. In Chapter 3 you will read about the five ways yang and yin uniquely express themselves in human beings. These two forms of *ki* create flows of energy through the body and rings of coincidence between the body and the physical, mental, emotional, and spiritual world outside it. These rings of earth, water, wood, fire, and metal reconnect the human body and human spirit to the greater world and give emotions, colors, seasons, sounds, smells, tastes, and symbols meaning in health.

Part 2 of this book is a snapshot of the home medicine cabinet of Kampo. The herbal formulas of Kampo are the means by which Japanese medicine restores balance to *ki*. They are also the means by which Japanese medicine, both traditional and modern, stops the symptoms of many diseases. These thirty-six herbal formulas are available as tablets or instant teas from grocers, health-food stores, pharmacies, and Asian medicine practitioners across the United States and Canada.

The formulas in Part 2 of this book are an essential sample of what the ancient Japanese referred to as "high-class medicine." They are safe, effective, and useful in treating not just one but many diseases. In the alphabetical listing of formulas in part two, you will find an explanation of each formula as energy medicine. They are described in the same terms as would be used by an acupuncturist or traditional Asian herbalist. You will also find an explanation of each formula as scientific medicine, described in terms of pharmacology, physiology, and modern medical practice.

Part 3 of this book presents the remainder of the eighty-four basic formulas of Kampo available in North America. Like the formulas in part two, these patent medicines are safe, effective, and manufactured under exacting standards of purity and quality. The difference is that these formulas are applicable to combinations of symptoms that are less frequently encountered. While these formulas do not belong in everyone's herbal medicine cabinet, they can be extraordinarily useful in treating specific diseases. Following the same pattern as Part 2, you will find an abbreviated explanation of each formula as energy medicine and scientific medicine, tested in laboratory and clinical trials.

The enlightened national health-care system of Japan pays for herbal formulas along with every other kind of medication, and so there is vast experience in using Kampo with, rather than against, modern medicine. In Japan, simply feeling "cold," that is, not having any symptoms but feeling run down, is considered a legitimate reason to consult a physician. To prevent vague symptoms from becoming serious ones, a Japanese physician is likely to prescribe one of the herbal formulas listed in this book. For everyday complaints, the healthiest nation on earth prefers Kampo.

It is important to remember, however, that while all but one formula in this book is suitable for self-treatment of illness, no formula in this book is intended to justify self-diagnosis regarding a serious illness. As a rule of thumb, any illness that causes acute and unbearable discomfort, or any illness that disrupts your daily routine for more than a month, calls for a medical examination. Then, when you have a diagnosis of your condition, use the formulas in this book to minimize your symptoms, accelerate your healing, and find a new level of health.

Introduction

Could there be anything new to write about herbs? Could there possibly be any new herbs to write about?

There is, and there are. This is a book about ancient Asian medicines newly arrived in the United States and Canada in their twenty-first-century form. These are the Japanese herbal formulas known as Kampo. Used in traditional healing for nearly two thousand years, these venerable natural treatments are now available as patent medicines. They provide standardized quality in tablets, powders, and instant drinks. Combining two to twenty herbs to correct a single set of symptoms, these eighty-four herbal patent medicine formulas are, for most people in North America, eighty-four new herbal combinations to treat disease, eighty-four new tools of natural healing.

Kampo products are FDA-approved for purchase without a prescription for self-treatment of virtually every common condition, from acne to yeast infections. This book presents the most important herbal combinations in traditional Asian medicine, available as effective, easy-to-use, and scientifically tested patent medicines. And while Kampo patent medicines are safe enough to be sold over the counter, they are potent enough to be used in the medically directed treatment of life-threatening conditions. Kampo is used to treat asthma, cancer, lupus, stroke, and hepatitis C. Kampo is employed in the treatment of these and other serious conditions in leading hospitals and research institutions, not only in Japan but also in the United States.

While every herb in Kampo medicine was first used in China, the distinguishing feature of these patent medicines made in Japan is their exceptional purity. Japanese patent medicines provide known herbs of reliable quality. The content of key ingredients in every capsule is standardized to hundredths of a milligram. The potency of key ingredients is expected to vary no more than a few tenths of a percent, even if the formula is stored for one, two, or as long as three years.

Like their Chinese counterparts, Japanese patent medicines are based on combinations of herbs rather than a single herb or nutrient. Every Kampo medicine contains two to twenty herbs. Each herb in turn provides literally dozens of phytochemical nutrients.

While one or two herbs are usually key to the healing process, additional herbs are almost always added to round out the formula. These secondary herbs eliminate potential side effects. They increase the amount of healing substances released by the formula into the digestive tract. They ease the absorption of key compounds into the body. They extend the healing process through multiple organ systems. By combining multiple herbs, Japanese herbal medicines provide a balanced healing effect that is both effective and economical. Chosen with care, a Kampo formula can replace some of the other nutritional supplements health-conscious consumers commonly take, at a fraction of their cost.

This book explains herbal formulas that are made in Japan, but no product described in this book is uniquely or even originally Japanese. Herbal medicines of all kinds are produced throughout Asia, but each tradition places a different emphasis on form. The healing traditions of Unani and Ayurveda in Iran and India do not exclude prescribed patent medicines, but they emphasize herbs used in combination with food. Nearly every community in China has a stock of herbal patent medicines for self-care. Chinese physicians, however, prefer to create complex combinations of herbs unique to each patient, to be prepared as teas. The teas are usually taken along with chemical pharmaceutical drugs. Korean consumers prefer to have their herbal teas brewed by the herbalist, and take home bottles of prescribed herbal tea for refrigeration and later use. Finely chopped herbs in tea bags and ready-made bottled teas are also available in Japan, but the Japanese generally prefer their herbs as tablets or powdered instant teas, which their physicians prescribe (and their health plans reimburse) as part of their primary care.

Consumer demand for easy-to-use herbal remedies in Japan, willingness of doctors to prescribe them, and coverage by health insurance plans to pay for them, has made Japan a leader in scientific herbal medicine. Herbal medicines provide exactly the same herbs with exactly the same chemical constituents, no matter which Japanese manufacturer makes them. These products can be scientifically scrutinized. As a result, Kampo medicines in Japan are beginning to undergo the same kinds of testing as prescription medicines in the United States. Used for thousands of years, these herbal formulas are assumed to be safe when given to people who meet the traditional "indications" for treatment. What the last thirty years of scientific testing has confirmed are the ways and means through which these ancient formulas change physiology and create well being.

No nation on earth enjoys a greater life expectancy than Japan, and the overwhelming majority of Japanese use Kampo medicine. The safe and effective patent medicines of Kampo are now on their way to physicians, hospitals, and pharmacies, to herbalists, naturopaths, and other natural healers, and to health-food stores, groceries, and supermarkets near you. Read this book to learn how to choose the right Kampo medicine for your condition, to bring you to a new state of good health simply, quickly, safely, and inexpensively.

Part I

和漢薬

The Theory of the Five Rings

Chapter 1

The Buddha, the Tiger, and the Scientist

Do you need something from outside yourself to be healthy? Or is everything you need to be healthy already inside you, only waiting to be released?

The fact is that all of us need resources both from outside ourselves and from within ourselves to be healthy. The difference between healing from without and healing from within is the fundamental distinction between the healing approaches of East and West.

Modern Western medicine excels at providing the tools of treatment to sick people. The scientifically trained physician zeroes in on the fundamental nature of an illness in order to repair a diseased organism. Any patient who presents a precise combination of symptoms has a specific illness, and any diagnosable illness can usually be treated in any of a number of ways. When the cause of the illness is known, Western medicine then uses every tool at its disposal to change, control, or destroy it. Even the basic tools of modern Western medicine are complex and can only be used by professionals.

Traditional East Asian medicine excels at uncovering the inner strengths of sick people to become well. The energy-savvy herbalist attunes herself to the fundamental nature of the patient in order to correct a unique imbalance. A patient who presents a known combination of symptoms can have any of a number of illnesses, but every combination of symptoms has a precise cure. When the energy imbalance affecting the person is recognized, traditional East Asian medicine then uses the single best herbal tool at its disposal to correct it. Even the advanced tools of modern East Asian herbal medicine are simple and can be used by anyone.

In many situations, Western medicine is the best medicine. I myself, for instance, only survive from day to day by the intervention of Western medicine. I have insulin-dependent diabetes. Years ago, most of the insulin-producing beta cells of my pancreas were destroyed by a viral infection, and my doctors' and my own mismanagement of the early stages of the disease finished off the rest of them. Since that time, I have had to take four injections of insulin a day, every day, without fail and without delay, to stay healthy and to stay alive.

I have to interrupt my activities several times a day to manage my blood sugars. I prick my finger, squeeze out a blood sample on a test strip, and place the test strip in a meter. Then I read a number from the meter to choose the appropriate number of units of insulin I need to inject into my bloodstream to bring my blood sugars to another, "healthy" number. Traditional East Asian medicine offers no alternatives to the insulin I require to continue life.

Traditional East Asian medicine offers numerous alternatives, however, for achieving health despite underlying illness. My personal epiphany regarding the use of herbal medicine took place over stages, but I became a convinced consumer of Japanese herbal medicine when I began to suffer some complications of long-term diabetes. At one point I developed a condition called neuropathy. I lost my normal sense of touch in my hands and feet, but they hurt nearly 24 hours a day. I could not walk across a room without considerable pain. I could not type at a computer keyboard for more than a few minutes at a time.

Then the neuropathy spread to other areas of my body. I could not sleep under a blanket, then under a sheet, and in a few weeks, I could scarcely sleep at all. The doctor offered me an antidepressant, which only changed my attitude toward my pain. Finally remembering that I could take Japanese herbal medicine, I chose a formula (Coptis Antidote, described on page 238) that gave me relief of symptoms within a week. These symptoms of neuropathy have never returned. Nonetheless, I still must take insulin every day.

My experience with the limitations of Western medicine is no different from the experience of tens of millions of people, possibly no different from your own. Western medicine is unquestionably the preferred approach to health conditions that have a simple, well-defined cause and effect like hitting your toe with a sledgehammer. It is the best medicine for conditions in which the body completely fails to make a vital substance, like insulin-dependent diabetes, although not necessarily for their complications. It is the best medicine for any condition in which the extent of the disease can be precisely measured. It is unquestionably the only rational approach to the emergency treatment of serious physical injuries. The public health and sanitation practices encouraged by Western medicine have banished infectious diseases and increased longevity around the globe.

For the conditions most of us have to deal with day by day, however, Western medicine suffers serious limitations. Common conditions tend to have multiple causes. The causes of disease may operate either independently or in combination. A headache can be due to fluid deprivation, or low blood sugars, or the early stages of an infection, among dozens of other etiologies. Heartburn can be symptomatic of a bacterial growth in the stomach, or a viral infection, or emotional stress. Quite frequently, heartburn is a side effect of inappropriate medication.

Western doctors and Western patients alike tend to treat "fuzzy" diseases as if they had a precise cause and a precise treatment. The problem with this approach is that the precise treatments for poorly defined conditions tend to have side effects. Suppose you have a headache caused by low blood sugars. The easiest treatment, which your doctor would recommend you take and call him in the morning, would be an aspirin.

You take the aspirin, and your headache disappears. Unfortunately, you haven't eaten, so the aspirin gives you heartburn. You then take a common medication for heartburn, which as a side effect gives you a headache. When the headache caused by the gastric histamine receptor-agonist you took wears off, you still have not eaten, so your hypoglycemic headache returns.

You have diagnosed yourself correctly, and you have taken an appropriate medication. Nonetheless, you suffer side effects, one of the side effects being the condition for which you took medication in the first place. In addition, since you did not treat the underlying cause of your symptoms, when the medicine that gave you your troublesome side effects wears off, your symptoms return.

More often than not, side effects are not so great that a medication cannot be taken. But also more often than not, unpleasant side effects occur when medication is taken.

In this regard, Kampo medicine is truly alternative. Traditional East Asian medicine tries to "zoom out" to the broadest possible understanding of a person to change an illness. Two patients who have the same symptoms may have entirely different illnesses, and two different illnesses may result in the same symptoms. No single symptom can define either an illness or a patient. The ability to respond to a disease with symptoms—with pain, with inflammation, with fever, with irritation or anxiety or even with hypochondria—is seen as a sign of the inner strength and resilience of the patient. The Japanese language even has a term for conditions that bring out the inner strengths of patients so that symptoms are obscure: *jitsuyu koho kampo* (with the kanji characters for this kampo different from the characters used for the herbal medicine Kampo), or "diseases that are not diseases."

The task of traditional East Asian medicine is to bring about a cure, by restoring harmony to the physical, emotional, and spiritual energies of the person. When harmony is restored, the health within the person becomes evident.

In this tradition of healing, one condition is treated with any of several medicines. This is true of headaches, for example. A headache accompanied by stomach upset would be treated with herbs that are entirely different from those used to treat a headache without stomach upset. A headache caused by low blood sugar would be treated by a formula that contains, among other ingredients, malt sugar. Individual differences are key to choosing treatments.

A more dramatic example of the radical difference between the approaches of West and East can be found in how they treat the most common health problem in the English-speaking countries: obesity. In Western medicine, the diagnosis of obesity is entirely objective. People who are sufficiently fat are obese. There are no individual differences, and all cases of obesity are the same.

In every case of obesity, in the eyes of Western medicine, the patient has failed to maintain normal weight. Therefore, the doctor's guidance is called for. The sole objective of treatment is to weigh less. Diet and exercise accomplish this. They are followed, in more difficult cases, by prescription drugs. Any subsequent weight loss is the success of medical advice, and any subsequent failure to lose weight (or gaining more weight!) is the patient's fault.

In the most severe cases of excess fat, the patient may be given prescription drugs or wheeled into surgery with potent, and sometimes tragic, side effects. But the only measure of success is to weigh less on the scales, and there is no help for you if you choose to continue to live as you are.

In healing traditions of China, Korea, and Japan, it is possible to make a diagnosis of obesity. However, there are no numerical charts, and no scales. In East Asian medicine, the diagnosis of obesity is largely subjective. Excess fat may be "hard" or "soft." "Hard" obesity is one among many symptoms of a vigorous, active individual whose underlying disharmony may be a tendency to "block" energies. These blocked energies may take the form of high blood pressure, headache, redness of the face, or excess weight.

Weight control is only part of a broader plan to get the body back into balance. First, herbs are administered to calm the metabolism and redirect energies. Only secondarily are there changes in diet and exercise. Success is recognized by the disappearance of blocked energies in all their manifestations, including but not limited to the disappearance of excessive fat.

"Soft" obesity is one of many symptoms in an individual in whom long-term stress has depleted the body's ability to maintain a normal form. Over a period of years, a vigorous person who once had a "hard" form of overweight can become fatigued. Muscles loosen. Skin sags. There may be recurrent infections, chronic fatigue, or weaknesses of hearing, sight, taste, or smell.

For the individual suffering "soft" obesity, treatment once again begins with herbs, but this time herbs are chosen which revitalize the metabolism and stimulate energies. Secondarily, there may be changes in diet or exercise. Success is recognized when the patient becomes more energetic and the symptoms of chronically depleted vitality begin to disappear. While weight loss is expected, it is not the only measure of success.

With such very different views of people, their health conditions, and the causes of illness, it is natural that practitioners of Western medicine and practitioners of East Asian medicine are usually at odds. One form of East Asian medicine, however, bridges both ways of thinking. This is the modern, yet ancient, form of herbal medicine from Japan known as Kampo.

Through much of the twentieth century, Japan followed the tenets of scientific medicine more fervently than any other nation in Asia. Japan's devotion to chemical healing methods began shortly after the Meiji Restoration in the middle of the nineteenth century. It continued into the first forty-five years of the twentieth century. As early as the 1870s, Japan enlisted Western physicians as consultants to its military efforts. Modern, Western, chemically driven medicine was thought to be essential to Japan's efforts to modernize. By 1912, Kampo medicine had been officially deemed a form of "folk" medicine that did not best serve the interests of the Empire.

Throughout this time, however, the Kampo tradition survived. A few herbal medicine societies, the herb vendors of the Doshomachi district in Osaka (about whom you will read more later in this chapter), and a few herb-oriented physicians continued to work quietly. One of these physicians, Keisetsu Otsuka, catalogued over 3,000 cases in both Western and traditional terms. He created a Rosetta Stone by which the terms of traditional East Asian medicine could be translated into the precise clinical diagnoses of Western medicine.

After World War II, the central government of Japan was greatly liberalized. The Japanese Ministry of Health established a national health-care system based on Western medicine. Responding to the popularity of the work of Keisetsu Otsuka and the efforts of many concerned herbal physicians, it also began to recognize and pay for herbal medicine. By 1990, medical schools had begun to offer courses in traditional herbalism and 148 herbal formulas were covered by health insurance and available to anyone. The nationwide acceptance of herbal medicine allowed thousands of doctors to gain experience with millions of patients, and to begin to publish their findings not only in Japanese but, more recently, and to a very limited extent, in English.

In the twenty-first century, Kampo medicine is both prescription medicine and over-the-counter medicine. Ready-made herb tablets and teas are available to everyone in Japan, not only from doctors but also from traditional herbalists. Since these herbal formulas were included in the national health insurance plan in 1967, the people of Japan have become among the healthiest in the world. Nowhere else on earth do both men and women live longer than in Japan, and, despite the fact nearly everyone lives within walking distance of a McDonald's, a Denny's, a Kentucky Fried Chicken, or at least a hot dog stand, in no industrialized country do fewer people suffer heart disease or cancer, or many of the diseases of aging.

The unsurpassed health of the Japanese people is quite possibly due to the fact that they are treated with the highest standards of medical care as well as the highest standards of herbal care. The modern medical method in Japan seeks to quell disease with resources external to the body. The ancient herbal healing tradition of Japan seeks to invigorate the internal, vital energies of life. For all of Japan's history, however, its traditional system of herbal medicine has had to adapt to survive, under the emblems of the Buddha, the tiger, and the scientist.

The Buddha

Hundreds of millions of people across the world agree that herbal medicine is a fountain of health. The freedom to take herbal medicine, however, is not universal and has not always existed. This is true even in the cultures that gave the world its best-known herbal healing traditions—India, China, and Japan. For most of their histories, herbs were not available to everyone. Doctors made herbs and other treatments available only to the royal family, military leaders, and the very wealthy. Common people were allowed exorcism and prayer.

Chinese herbal medicine was first brought to Japan in 562, when a young Chinese Buddhist monk named Zhi Cong arrived in Japan carrying textbooks. These textbooks included the *Yellow Emperor's Classic of Internal Medicine*, as well as the sacred texts of Buddhism. The techniques of Kampo medicine made a favorable impression on the royal court of the Empress Suiko, who sent for Chinese physicians to treat her husband in 587. However, the missionary monk was more concerned for the spiritual state of the royal family than for their physical health.

For Zhi Cong, medicine was just one of the gifts of Buddha. Millenniums before medicine of any sort was practiced in Japan, herbal medicine had been known in both India, the birthplace of the Buddha, and in China, where Buddhism took hold. Zhi Cong taught that this form of healing was a gift of the Bhaisajya-Guru, a buddha who offers medicine to people suffering from illness and who grants nourishment to both the mind and body. This buddha, also known as the Guru of Emerald Radiance, held a container holding all kinds of medicines in his left hand. He blessed the vows made by the faithful with his right hand.

Bhaisajya-Guru bore gifts that contrasted with those of the Amida Buddha, who presided over the Western Pure Land of future rebirths. Known in Japanese as Yakushi Nyorai, the Emerald Buddha granted practical benefits in the present life as Lord of the Eastern Pure Land. Japanese Buddhist priests came to take for granted that the Eastern Pure Land was Japan.

Two hundred years after the work of the Buddhist missionary, the Emperor Shonmu called on his subjects to pray to Buddha for the recovery of his wife. The emperor's wife in fact recovered and became the Empress Komyo. In 747 she consecrated the temple of Yakushi-ji, a shrine to the Medicine Buddha. Her successor, Empress Komyo, likewise prayed to the Medicine Buddha for the healing of her husband, Emperor Shomu. When her prayers were answered, she commissioned the building of Shin-Yakushi-ji, a play on words that means both "new temple of Yakushi-ji" and "wonder-working temple of Yakushi-ji." This sanctuary was dedicated in 747.

For centuries after the first introduction of herbal medicine, the prescribed rule of Japanese medicine was to pray to the Medicine Buddha for healing. Herbs were only dispensed by Buddhist priests, whose first priority was the continuation of the practice of prayer. It was not until 1536 that Kampo medicines became available to anyone who wished to buy them, at least in the Doshomachi district in the coastal fishing village that was later to be known as Osaka.

The beginning of the sixteenth century had brought a brief time in which Japan was extraordinarily open to the world. Dutch traders brought both European goods and European medicines to Japan's trading centers. While Chinese medicine had been available to the imperial family for nearly 1,000 years, this was the first time in Japan's history that herbal medicines were available to common people other than as gifts from priests. A guild of herb vendors organized in Osaka, where trade in the herbal medicines they called Kampo flourished.

Kampo medicine was clearly understood to be Chinese medicine.

The word Kampo is the Japanese pronunciation of a combination of two Chinese characters: *Kan*, or *Han*, which means "from China," and *po*, or *ho*, which means "way" or "law." The term "Kampo" is an easier and accepted way of pronouncing "Kanpo."

As Japan's "Chinese way" to health and healing, all of the herbal formulas used in Kampo had the same historical sources as their counterparts in Traditional Chinese Medicine (TCM). These formulas had been recorded verbatim in the *Ishimpo*, a medical encyclopedia of thirty volumes presented to the imperial court in 984. The term Kampo, however, only became common in the Japanese language after a new system of medicine was brought to Japan from Europe. This was called *Rampo* ("Dutch medicine"), because the Dutch first introduced it. In order to distinguish it from the newly introduced European-style medicine, the indigenous medicine came to be called *Kampo*, or medicine from China.

Only a century after Dutch medicine arrived, however, selling foreign medicines became a politically sensitive activity. In 1633, the shogun Iemitsu forbade travel abroad. In 1639 he almost completely isolated Japan by reducing contacts with the outside world to very limited trade relations with China and the Netherlands in the port of Nagasaki. In addition, any possession of foreign books was banned under penalty of death. The *Ishimpo* record of the classic formulas of Chinese medicine was considered a Japanese book, but the Chinese books brought to Osaka in the sixteenth century had to be burned. And since the formulas of Kampo were based on the classic books of Chinese medicine, it became necessary to remember the gift of the Buddha in a very different way.

Prior to the closure of Japan to the outside world, the fact that Kampo medicines were based on the teachings of the ancient Chinese masters brought prestige to the herb vendors of Doshomachi. With the new laws, however, a new authority was required. The story of Japanese medicine was then remembered as founded to preserve "laws" given to the peoples of Asia by the Buddha himself.

While this retelling of the origins of Kampo medicine sufficed during the reign of the shogun Iemitsu, a later shogun enlisted scholars to write a comprehensive history of Japan. The telling of the origins of herbal medicine in Japan, of course, then had to be made consistent with the *Kojiki*, the official record of the history of Japan. Kaibara Ekiken (1630-1714), author of the *Yamata Honso (The Herbal Reference of Japan)* retold the story of the origins of Japanese, and, within his frame of reference, all medicine, in terms of the Shinto religion.

In Ekiken's story, the creator deity Musubi-no-kami entrusted Japan to his eight sons. One of these sons, Ohkuni-nushi-no-mikoto, whose name is approximately translated as "Prince of Izumo," was master first of peach blossoms and then of all of agriculture. The storyteller said that the Prince of Izumo was blessed with a gentle disposition from birth, and enjoyed the warm trust of his people. He displayed great skill in the management of his land, so that even in cold years with much rainfall, even when Japan was visited by raging typhoons, and even in droughts caused by rainless summers, he always had plenty of grain in reserve to protect his people from want.

One day, as the Prince of Izumo was touring the countryside to give guidance to the farmers, a ship appeared on the horizon. The boat had a mirror attached to its bow. In the boat was a man no one recognized, until a woman named Kuyehiko came forward and said, "That is Sukuna-Hikona, the worthless remainder of the fifteen-hundred children of Kanmimusubi (a less learned term for the creator deity), one who slipped through the fingers that were counting." Sukuna-hikona-no-mikoto, however was not a "worthless remainder" but a "saving grace." Another son of the creator deity, Prince Sukuna-Hikona, had been dispatched in his youth to take enlightenment to India and China, but had returned to rule over Japan with his brothers. He brought back to Japan his special knowledge of herbal healing.

Sukuna-hikona-no-mikoto joined forces with his brother Ohkuni-nushi-no-mikoto to make special efforts to look after the physical health of people and animals. They exploited new herbs to remove both physical and spiritual suffering. They cured illnesses of both people and animals with kindness and loving care.

In the age in which the gods were physically present in Japan, there was need to write down prescriptions. The marvelously effective medicines of their time reflected the divine virtue of the two gods. By the time of the historian Kaibara Ekiken in the seventeenth century, however, the gods had left Japan. Fortunately, Sukuna-hikona-no-mikoto had done missionary work among the Chinese, who had recorded his herbal prescriptions before he returned to Japan.

The Tiger

Unfortunately, Sukuna-hikona-no-mikoto did not record his herbal prescriptions in Osaka. The great books of Japanese herbal medicine were all kept at the imperial offices in Edo. All the telling and retelling of the myth of Kampo led the herb vendors of Doshomachi simply to sell the herbal combinations they wanted without any reference to their authenticity. Profitability replaced accountability, and cheap medicines made from whatever herbs were available became the norm. Kampo medicine became less and less authentically Chinese among the herb vendors through the reigns of seven shoguns, until in 1722 the eighth shogun, Tokugawa Yoshimune, fell ill in Osaka while on a trip.

In early Japan, as in China, the task of the imperial physician had been to keep the emperor well. When the emperor fell ill, he was likely to have his physician beheaded. The one 124 Kampo pharmacists treating the emperor therefore decided it would be wise to use the formulas of the Chinese masters.

Fortunately for the herbalists, the herbs they gave their shogun resulted in an almost immediate cure. When the shogun returned to his palace, he issued an edict licensing the 124 herbalists of Doshomachi as official purveyors of herbal medicine. At the same time, he protected them from competition by establishing an Imperial Herbal Quality Center, charging the herb vendors to be sure of the quality of their products, since a single misidentified herb could cost a life.

Official recognition that herbs could be harmful as well as helpful put the herb vendors in a difficult position. They now could draw on the knowledge of Chinese medicine that had survived since the beginning of Japan's isolation, but they needed to be able to credit, or blame, a uniquely Japanese deity for its results. At first, the herbalists' guild founded a "prayer circle" for divine protection and to ensure the safety and efficacy of their formulas. Then in 1780 the guild founded a shrine to house the divine spirit of Sukuna-hikona-no-mikoto, inviting him to leave his shrine in Kyoto to join the local medical deity Shinno.

Despite the guild's devotion to Sukuna-hikona-no-mikoto, the one-hundredth anniversary of its founding brought disaster. In the summer of 1822 Osaka was struck by an epidemic of cholera. This plague most likely was brought by traders who had ventured, whether legally or not, to China and returned to Osaka rather than to the official port city of Nagasaki. Since cholera was an infection spread from nation to nation by sailing ships, Japan had never experienced the disease. And since cholera was essentially unknown in East Asia before 1817, there were no ancient herbal formulas on which to rely.

The herbalists of Doshomachi worked feverishly to find a treatment. The only guidance from the ancient masters was that general weakness called for tiger bone, the strongest part of the strongest animal. The herbalists therefore worked out a treatment, *koto-sakkiyuoen,* or Tiger Pill, which included powdered tiger bones.

Fewer than one in twenty people who took the pill suffered serious symptoms. Almost everyone quickly recovered. What the herbalists could not have known was that, even with no treatment, only about one person in twenty who is infected with cholera suffers life-threatening symptoms, and the majority recover with minimal treatment. Nonetheless, Tiger Pill was pronounced marvelously effective and demand quickly surpassed supply.

The herbalists were faced with a second dilemma. They had been charged by the emperor himself to provide only medicines of known purity. They could not sell a placebo. Accordingly, they did the next best thing: they had artisans craft tens of thousands of papier-maché tigers to be distributed as protective amulets throughout the city.

The paper tigers proved every bit as effective as the Tiger Pill. Throughout Osaka, almost everyone was spared the dreadful new disease. And while the pharmacological efficacy of the Tiger Pill is questionable, the provision of tigers made of papier-maché marked a rare accomplishment in the history of herbal medicine. Even in the prospect of enormous profits, the herbalists of Doshomachi had declined to sell a product with a falsified list of ingredients. And when the Tokugawa period ended in 1868, the guild returned to the precise use of the ancient Chinese herbal formulas.

The herbal guild of Doshomachi survived the introduction of Western medicine and the wars of the twentieth century. And even in the twenty-first century, the herbalists of Doshomachi still distribute paper tigers at an annual festival of the Shinno Shrine every November 22 and 23. A tradition of honesty concerning the products it sells and its exacting faithfulness to the formulas of the ancient Chinese masters have enabled Japan to become a center of scientific herbal medicine.

The Scientist

Kampo formulas have been used by tens of millions of people for hundreds of years. Their safety is obvious. However, their effectiveness in terms of modern medicine has to be determined through scientific testing.

Prior to 1960, rigorous scientific testing of drugs of any sort was not the norm in either Japan or the United States. If patients received a treatment and got better, their improvement was assumed to be due to the treatment. Since Kampo formulas had been making people better for centuries, they were assumed to be effective.

In the United States, however, there was a strong movement toward a more "scientific" model. The use of control or placebo groups and treatment groups allowed the use of inferential statistics, in which less experience with healing—that is, treating hundreds of patients in a study lasting a year rather than treating millions of patients over the course of centuries—allowed the estimation of probabilities of success. The numbers of patients getting better in the placebo and control groups of rigorously designed clinical experiments were counted and compared. If more patients got better in the test group than in the placebo group, their numbers were compared.

Inferential statistics allowed an estimate of the probability that the measured change in patients was due to the tested drug. A probability or "p value" of .95 or .99 or .999 meant that, under the conditions of the study, there was a 95 percent or 99 percent or 99.9 percent chance that any change in the patient was associated with the treatment. If statistical analysis yielded a sufficiently high "p value," the treatment became medically accepted.

The scientific model is most easily applied to the study of a single treatment affecting a single process of a single disease. Therefore, therapies that were based on chemicals, studied in the laboratory, and influenced a specific, isolated, precisely measured healing process became privileged in Western medicine. The herbal remedies that once made up virtually all of a Western doctor's healing repertoire were eliminated from mainstream medical practice.

The scientific model slowly permeated American medicine. By 1990, it had become impossible to get government grants to do medical research under any other approach.

By and large, the nations of Asia have been slow to adopt the scientific model of medical research. This is not the case, however, in Japan. The scientific investigation of Kampo is an enormous enterprise in Japan. There are academic departments for the study of Japanese herbal medicine at Toyama Medical and Pharmaceutical University, Kinki University, Tokyo Women's Medical College, the Tsumura Institute for the Study of Oriental Medicine at the School of Medicine at Keio University, and the Oriental Medicine Research Center at the Kitasato Institute. Over 10,000 physicians and scientists are engaged in research in Kampo medicine through the Japan Oriental Medicine

Society. Over 1,200 scientists are members of the Medical and Pharmaceutical Society for Wakan-Yaku (Japanese traditional medicine). Research on medicinal plants, natural substance chemistry, cultivation and production of medicinal plants and traditional medicine, and development of new drugs of plant origin, is the concern of the 1,428 members of the Japan Society for Pharmacognosy, and 1,800 physicians and pharmacists are members of The Association for East-Asian Medicine.

The advantage of Kampo is that every manufacturer uses exactly the same herbs in exactly the same amount to make any given formula. This reliability makes it possible to test the effects of the formula on the absorption of prescription drugs, or to explain the action of the formula in physiological terms, or to test the formula in clinical trials. While not every Kampo formula has received any of the kind of testing done in the United States on prescription drugs, over 30 have, and these formulas contain combinations of herbs that are found in the other 180 herbal formulas that are commonly used in Japan.

But Kampo is also faithful to the principles of Asian medicine. As you will see in the following chapters, the formulas that are valid in science are also valid for manipulating Yang and Yin and the vital energy *ki*.

Chapter 2

Herbal Medicine as a Martial Art

Herbal medicine was introduced to Japan as a martial art. In the year 562 a Chinese Buddhist monk named Zhi Cong arrived at the Imperial Court. He brought with him the source books of his faith. He carried the codes of law that were to become the *Taiho Ryo-ritsu*, the Great Treasure Code. This was the legal reference that was to become the organizing principle of future Japanese governments.

Zhi Cong probably also introduced Japan to Chinese pastimes, such as kites and board games, including an early version of Chinese checkers. And he brought 160 medical books, among them the esteemed textbook of medicine, the *Huang-di Nei-Jing*. This book is also known as the *Yellow Emperor's Classic of Internal Medicine*.

The *Nei-Jing*, dating from 170 B.C., was the oldest textbook of medicine in China. It is thought to be the first textbook of medicine written in the history of the world. However, it was (and is) considered unclear, inconsistent, written in obscure terminology, and appropriate only for the most advanced students of herbal medicine. Since Japan had no students of medicine at all, the *Yellow Emperor's Classic* received little attention in the royal court. Instead, a more accessible book, written in the terminology of the martial arts, became the foundation of Japanese herbal medicine. This book was the *Shang Han Lun*, or the *Discussion of Infectious Cold*, written shortly after 200 A.D. by the venerable physician Zhang Zhong-jing.

The doctor Zhang had lived in the eastern realm of the Han Empire in the city of Luo yang. The second and third centuries A.D. were a time of political turmoil and rampant epidemics. For one hundred and fifty years China had been ruled by teenage emperors. The imperial court had placed the day-to-day affairs of the Han Empire in the hands of advisors. The political establishment encouraged these boy kings to lead lives of sexual excess and drunkenness that invariably led to early death, thereby ensuring the continuation of the advisors in power.

The court physician, of course, had a very easy job. Since the emperor's illness and early death was desired by those who actually held power, the practice of medicine became a farce. Eventually the royal advisors themselves abandoned sensible health practices. A chronicle of the history of China recorded that in about 170 A.D. a young Dr. Zhang had an audience with the privy secretary, who that year was over twenty. The *Zhen Jiu Jia Yi Jing* records that Zhang told the minister, "Sire, you are sick. At the age of forty your hair will fall out and within half a year you will die. If you take Five Stones Herbal Formula now, you can avoid this." The minister refused to take the formula. Twenty years later the minister's hair did fall out, and on the 187th day thereafter, he died.

In about 190 A.D., unchecked by the royal court, the Imperial commander Dong Zhuo sacked and burned Zhang's home city. The general's plan was to destroy the capital, Luoyang, in order to concentrate his power in the western capital Changan. Not a single building was left standing. One history of the atrocity records that when General Dong was informed that the common people did not have even rats to eat, he replied, "What do I care of the common people when I can seize China?"

In the lawlessness and chaos that followed in the Eastern Kingdom, starvation and epidemics were rampant. The physician Zhang lost over 140 of his relatives to *shang han*, a condition that most likely should translated as "infectious cold." The impotence of doctors to help his relatives infuriated Zhang, and inspired him to write a new textbook of medicine.

In his preface Zhang railed against the foppish doctors of the imperial court. "It is bewildering," Zhang wrote, "that the learned men of our age never pay attention to medicine and are not proficiently versed in the healing arts, which would enable them to treat the illnesses of the sovereign and of their elders above, to relieve the suffering of the poor and destitute below, and to safeguard their own body and sustain health at its center, all in order to cultivate life. Instead, they only compete to pursue glory and power. They stand on the tiptoe of expectancy for influential officials and families of power, diligently and untiringly devoting their efforts only to fame and profit. Revering and refining nonessentials, they neglect the root." Having forgotten herbal medicine, the doctors of Zhang's time gave themselves over to witchcraft. "Abandoning their integrity, they lower themselves to grovel before magical healers," Zhang continued sardonically. "Declaring their helplessness, they attribute their misfortune to fate ordained by heaven . . . The body already dead and the spirit destroyed, they transmute into weird beings."

While the doctors of the court could recite the *Yellow Emperor's Classic* and gave learned explanations of the vital life force *ki*, their understanding of the energies of life had become entirely mysterious. They had forgotten practical, herbal cures.

Zhang sought both to recover the medical knowledge that had been lost during the previous 150 years. He resolved to write a textbook of medicine that could be available to the common people. He also sought to appeal to the new military rulers of China by presenting a new model of infectious disease in familiar military terms.

Disease in Time and Space. The *Shang Han Lun* describes disease as a struggle of the body against outside pernicious evils. The idea of undesirable energies entering the body and causing disease was probably universally accepted in ancient East Asia, but other textbooks of medicine in Zhang's time described these pathological energies in puzzling terms. The aptly entitled *Book of Difficulties*, for instance, offered the opinion that "There are five types of cold damage. These are wind stroke, cold, damp warmth, heat disease, and warm disease."

Zhang described the invading energies of disease in clearer terms. Since the body is an earthly manifestation of heaven's warmth, Zhang reasoned, its most obvious enemy is cold. There were, of course, other commonsensical and obvious enemies of health. These included dampness, heat, and wind. The pernicious and pathological energy of disease of could be any force draining the energies of the body. In modern terms, these energy entities could correspond to a virus or a bacterium, an upsetting emotion, extremes of the environment, or an injury.

The *Yellow Emperor's Classic of Internal Medicine*, the bible of medicine for the imperial court of China, gave an elegant explanation of how pernicious evils overcame the body's immune defenses. On the first day of invading cold, the physicians to the Yellow Emperor are reported to have said, the pernicious evil injures the outermost energies of the body, the *Tai Yang*. On the second day of illness the evil cold injures the second layer of the energies of the body, the *Yang Ming*. On the third day it injures the *Shao Yang*, the fourth day the *Tai Yin*, the fifth day the *Shao Yin*, the sixth day the *Jue Yin*. (These names also refer to energy channels used in acupuncture, but the connection was not noted in Chinese medicine until more than 1,200 years after the time of the Yellow Emperor.) If the patient survived six days, the pattern repeated itself.

While this theory was adequate for the physicians to the boy emperors, for Zhang it held little value. The *Tai Yang*, *Yang Ming*, *Shao Yang*, *Tai Yin*, *Shao Yin*, and *Jue Yin* were only meaningless abstractions, and symptoms of disease certainly do not repeat themselves in a six-day cycle. For Zhang it was of primary importance to understand that different "layers" of the body could experience illness at different times, so that appropriate herbal remedies could be applied.

To explain the battle between illness and health, Zhang recovered a more ancient understanding of the concepts of Yang and Yin. Yang energies are aggressive. Yin energies are defensive.

The first three battlegrounds of the fight between the body and disease are found in the Yang energy layers. These house the outwardly directed energies of the body. The second three battlegrounds of the fight between the body and disease are found in the Yin energy layers. These house the containing energies of the body. Each level of energy disturbance produces particular symptoms, and each combination of symptoms can be corrected with an herbal formula. Since human anatomy was largely unknown, Zhang defined Yang and Yin in terms of energies and obvious symptoms, rather than in terms of the physical makeup of organs and tissues.

The energies of the *Tai Yang*, which is translated as "Greater Yang," were the most vigorous energies of immune response. This layer combated the earliest stages of disease. If the energies of the body were perfectly matched to the energies of the disease, the pathogen would be routed with no disturbance to the body and no symptoms. This, of course, is the normal condition of the body. Energy influences constantly come and go without disruption to body functions.

When a pernicious energy causes an imbalance in the Greater Yang, it protects the body with violent and visible symptoms. It produces fevers, rashes, or outbursts of emotion. In some instances, the Greater Yang "bottles up" the pathogen and forces it to starve, as in a tight neck containing tension. In other cases, the Greater Yang flushes out the pathogen through blood, sweat, vomit, or tears. It may torture the pathogen with fiery fever. If the pathogen does not flee out of the body or into a deeper layer of the body, the immune system destroys it.

The common element of all the reactions of the Greater Yang is that the body overreacts to an invading pernicious evil. It applies more energy than is needed to stop disease. This excess of energy produces any or all of a number of disagreeable symptoms. These include:

- Acute fever
- Chills

- Headache
- Painful tension of the neck and shoulder muscles
- Joint pain
- Muscle pain
- Stuffy nose
- Sore throat
- Inflammation of the upper respiratory system

Zhang's therapeutic principle for the First Stage of Disease was to "loosen up" the energy surface of the body. To accomplish this, he prescribed herbs that stimulate the circulation of blood and energy. These herbs "dissolve" cold trapped in this energy layer. To facilitate the dissolution of cold, Zhang ordered his patients to be confined to bed until sweating was observed.

Unlike his predecessors, Zhang offered precise combinations of herbs for precise combinations of symptoms. In fact, he referred to diseases by the herbs needed to treat them. An upset stomach might be a "cinnamon formula" disorder, or hepatitis might be a "minor bupleurum formula" disorder. Zhang recognized the right formula for a given pattern of symptoms by how "energized" the outer layers of the body appeared to be during the First Stage of Disease. If a patient in the First Stage of Disease was so "superheated" that there was no sweating, but suffered the wheezing and shortness of breath we associate with asthma, Zhang offered Ephedra Formula. If another "superheated" patient in the First Stage of Disease suffered especially severe pain due to tension of the neck and shoulder muscles, Zhang offered Kudzu Formula. If the Yang energies were milder and the patient was sweating, Zhang offered Minor Bluegreen Dragon Formula for runny nose. For the first time in medical history, Zhang categorized herbal remedies by the symptoms they treated.

Zhang solemnly charged his students not to apply herbs without close attention to the pattern of symptoms they were meant to treat, even when the patient was strong. A single instance of inappropriate treatment, he noted, will lengthen the time needed for recovery.

Further errors of treatment, even of patients in relatively vigorous health, could lead to death. These instructions were echoed in Doshomachi over 1,500 years later, in the shogun's establishment of a quality assurance center for the herbalists' guild.

Zhang applied the same principles to his prescriptions for the remaining five stages of disease. The Second Stage of Disease begins when the pathogen overwhelms the body's ability to produce strong, outwardly visible symptoms. The immune system continues to respond to the pathogen but with lesser force. The battle between the body and the outside pernicious influence is still at the level of the skin, the muscles, and the immune system, but the body's response is weaker and the chances of recovery are reduced. A respiratory infection that could only challenge the body to produce symptoms of a cold or hay fever in the First Stage of Disease challenges the body to produce the symptoms of bronchitis, asthma, or pneumonia in the Second Stage of Disease. Wheezing becomes shortness of breath. A sore throat becomes a lump in the throat. Sniffles become glutinous phlegm. Food poisoning that induced vomiting now only causes nausea. Zhang tailored herbal formulas to unique combinations of symptoms in the Second Stage of Disease, just he had for the first (see tables 2.1 and 2.2).

Table 2.1. Herbal Remedies for Distress in the Chest

Energy Status	Particular Symptoms	Herbal Remedy
Excessive energy expenditure in the chest	Coughing, perspiration, thirst, phlegm	Five Tiger Formula (page 245)
	Coughing, wheezing, fever, asthma in children	Mysterious Decoction (page 268)
Normal energy expenditure in the chest	Coughing, wheezing, feeling of lump in the throat.	Bupleurum and Magnolia Formula (page 122)
	Coughing, restlessness, feeling of lump in the throat	Pinellia and Magnolia bark Formula (page 272)
Deficient energy expenditure in the chest	Shortness of breath, easy fatigue, racing pulse	Honey-Fried Licorice Formula (page 261)
	Coughing, dry throat	Japanese Lily Formula (page 262)

Table 2.2 Herbal Remedies for Distress in Digestive Tract

Energy Status	Particular Symptoms	Herbal Remedy
Excessive energy expenditure in the digestive tract	Alternating depression and restlessness ("mood related to food") Constipation, tenderness on the right side of the abdomen, insomnia	Bupleurum, Dragon Bone, and Oyster Shell Formula (page 224) Major Bupleurum Formula (page 177)
Normal energy expenditure in the digestive tract	Abdominal pain, chest, congestion, feeling of heat in the upper part of the body Pain in the upper abdomen, soft stools, sound of rumbling in the stomach	Coptis Formula (page 238) Pinellia Draining Formula (page 274)
Deficient energy expenditure in the digestive tract	Vomiting, sweating, cramps, headache, abdominal tension Stress-induced stomach pain, sound of fluctuating liquid in the stomach, vomiting	Bupleurum and Cinnamon Formula (page 222) Two-Cured Formula (page 282)

If disease wins the fight in the Second Stage of Disease, the body must continue the battle at a still deeper level. Zhang believed that the Third Stage of Disease took place in the "Shadow Yang," where the body's immune resistance was a "shadow" of its former strength. When disease reached this level, Zhang thought, the body activated the fascia, tendons, ligaments, and bones. These organs actively fight disease, but at the cost of their ability to carry the body's internally generated energies to its surface, that is, to the skin and muscles.

The third layer of the body fights disease by increasing body temperature. Fever may be continuous, but the hands and feet are cold, showing the overall lack of defensive energy in the body. There may be constipation and thirst. The body lacks the energy to circulate fluids and blood. Blood accumulates in the body and creates a condition known in Japanese as *oketsu.*

The energy diagnosis of *oketsu* is very important to the modern, Japanese understanding of Zhang's Third Stage of Disease because it is an energy state that can be identified under a microscope. When patients show the classical symptoms of *oketsu* there are lesions of the endothelial cells lining the blood vessels and leaks of blood into surrounding tissues. Areas of tenderness on the abdomen associated with *oketsu* frequently correspond to displacements of internal organs that are visible on an X ray. Beyond the microscopic level, *oketsu* expresses itself as flush, muscle pain, lumbago, darkened pigment in the skin and circles under eyes, spasms of peripheral blood vessels, and painful hemorrhoids.

As bad as these symptoms are, in the Fourth Stage of Disease symptoms get worse. When disease overwhelms the third level of defensive energies, the body's strategy turns from offense to defense. Zhang considered the next three stages of disease to provoke the body's energies of Yin. Like Yang, Yin has many meanings in East Asian medicine. In this context, however, Yin only refers the body's ability to "contain" itself. The Yin keeps blood and fluids in their proper channels and enables the organs to maintain their normal shapes. Yin energy is essential to the body's ability to transform food into tissue and energy. When the body is under attack, however, it expends Yin to fight disease.

The Fourth Stage of Disease is called the Tai Yin, or Greater Yin. At this point the battle between the outside pernicious evil and the body is still focused in the fascia, tendons, ligaments, and bones, but the effort of the body is to maintain the normal shapes of tissues and organs and to keep blood and fluids flowing in their normal pathways. The overall energy of the body is deficient, and it desperately tries to maintain its form.

Therefore, in the fourth stage, the energies of Yin are excessive. Yin holds fluids where they do not belong, causing swelling, or it holds energies back from where they are needed, causing fatigue. The Yin energies of the digestive tract are redirected to other organs, so the digestive tract cannot hold food. The result is diarrhea, in which the stools contain partially digested food. As in the Lesser Yang, there may also be *oketsu,* or stagnant circulation. In this stage, however, stagnant blood is accompanied by a weakened heart and a slower pulse. The problems caused by the leakage of blood into tissues are compounded by generally poor circulation.

The Fourth Stage of Disease corresponds to many of the most troubling conditions of Western medicine. Alzheimer's disease, chronic gastritis, eczema, many kinds of menstrual irregularities, rheumatoid arthritis, and children's bedwetting are all manifestations of the Greater Yin. Once again, however, Zhang offered precise prescriptions to match the combinations of symptoms presented in this level of disease (see Table 2.3).

Table 2.3 Herbal Remedies for Symptoms of the Greater Yin

Energy Status	Particular Symptoms	Herbal Remedy
Body as whole has adequate energy, yin is excessive	Abdominal distention, bloat and gas, constipation, easy fatigue, stress-induced symptoms of the digestive tract	Cinnamon and Peony Formula (page 235)
	Colicky pain of the bile duckt, intestine, or urethra; "convulsive" lapses of consciousness	Rhubarb and Moutan Formula (page 279)
Body as whole has deficient energy, Yin is excessive	Abdominal pain, distress in the chest, with accumulation of fluid, nightsweats, fatigue, and/or eczema	Astragalus Formula (page 116)
	Tension in the neck, swelling, vertigo, alterations of consciousness similar to those of Alzheimers's disease	Dong Quai and Peony Formula (page 150)

In the Fifth Stage of Disease, the Shao Yin Lesser Yin, the body has even less Yin energy to fight off the pathogen. The internal organs—the heart, the lungs, the kidneys, the liver, and the intestines—begin to expend their energy to fight disease. Their needs outstrip the body's abilities to process nutrients, with the unhappy result that diarrhea becomes an even greater problem. The body can neither hold food nor extract its energy.

As immune energies become exhausted, the battle enters the Sixth Stage of Disease, the Absolute Yin. Recovery from this stage is unlikely. The symptoms of the Fifth and Sixth Stages of Disease correspond to the symptoms of pulmonary fibrosis, cirrhosis of the liver, collagen diseases, chronic renal failure, and the later stages of AIDS.

Even for these most serious diseases, Zhang offered treatment. These especially "cold" conditions required exceptionally "hot" (and potentially toxic) herbs. Some of Zhang's formulas for the Fifth and Sixth Stages of Disease are discussed in Part 2 of this book.

The Universal Duality. While Zhang saw Yang and Yin principally as the direction the body sent its energies to respond to disease, these concepts have a richer meaning that underlies the whole of East Asian medicine. Yang and Yin are universal characteristics of both ordinary matter and the vital energy *ki* (pronounced "kee" and corresponding to the Chinese *chi* or *qi*, both pronounced "chee"). Despite the importance of this term, none of the Oriental healing traditions offers a precision definition for it. For Western readers, the concept of *ki* itself requires examples and explanation.

Speakers of the Japanese language cannot avoid referring to the vital energy *ki*. This syllable and its associated kanji character are the root of over 100 words in Japanese. *Reiki* speaks of the universal life force and *kion* of temperature. The dynamic forces of the physical world possess *ki*, as is shown in the words *denki*, electricity; *tenki*, weather; and *kuki*, which refers to "no *ki*," or air.

Ki describes many human attributes. A formal greeting, *o-genki desu ka*, inquires about *genki*, the state of essential *ki*. The way one holds *ki* or the way one feels is known *kimochi*. A painful *kimochi* is a *kinodoku*, or an injury to one's *ki*. When something or somebody suits the distinctive Japanese taste, it is described as *ki ni iru*, which means it is "agreeable, suitable, acceptable." If something really catches a person's attention, a proper response is *ki ni narimashita*. A person who does not demonstrate an acceptable degree of goodwill, energy and spirit, especially in a work situation, causes his or her co-workers to feel *ki ni kuwanai*, or that person is "distasteful."

On a basic level, *ki* is the means by which the mind interacts with the physical world. The Japanese expression for giving a small gift translates as, "*Ki* (action) speaks for the heart." A small gift does not convey the whole of a person's feelings, but it does convey something of sentiment. Similarly, *ki* does not convey the whole of the mind, which exists both within and beyond the physical realm, but embodies its attitudes.

The two most important "attitudes" of *ki* are Yang and Yin. Over the past half-century, the terms Yang and Yin have entered the everyday vocabulary of the English language as key terms of East Asian philosophy. They are not only basic concepts of traditional Chinese, Japanese, and Korean philosophy, science, politics, and medicine. They are also the most basic concepts of East Asian thought. While using Kampo medicines requires no knowledge of East Asian thought at all, using Kampo in a traditional way requires at least an elementary understanding of this universal duality.

The earliest references to Yang and Yin appeared in the *Book of Changes* (the *I Ching*) about 2,700 years ago. In ancient China, entire universities devoted themselves to the philosophical study of just these two concepts. In terms of healing practice, a rough but useful explanation of Yang and Yin can be summarized in two sentences very similar to Zhang's understanding of the terms: Yang moves. Yin holds.

The Yellow Emperor's Classic of Internal Medicine explained Yang and Yin in cosmic terms. "Heaven is an accumulation of Yang," the Yellow Emperor is told, and "Earth is an accumulation of Yin." In its purest form, Yang is pure energy and Yin is pure matter. Yang produces energy, while Yin produces form. Yang generates, while Yin grows. Yang is speed, expansion, rising, and potential. Yin is caution, contraction, falling, and form. However, in East Asian philosophy, Yang and Yin are inseparable, opposite stages of an ever-repeating cycle of breaking down and building up.

Ancient Asian philosophers could see these opposing forces at work everywhere. The heat of Yang melted an ore to yield a metal. The cold of Yin allowed the flowing metal to fill a mold. The warm Yang of the morning sun dispersed the morning fog to the heavens. The cold Yin of night caused the fog to form.

In the case of the human body, however, Yang and Yin did not act so simply. The human body seemed to channel Yang and Yin according to human purposes. That is, outwardly directed Yang energies seem to flow in a certain direction through certain organs of the body, while the containing energies of Yin seemed to flow in the opposite direction through other organs of the body.

In an age of wild animals and marauding bandits, every person had to protect her back. The back, then, was recognized as the place where all the Yang energies flow. These channels carry Yang energy and protect the body from pathogenic organisms. Yang energy is also the carrier of outward expression, rising to the face and head. The Yang energies of the environment, such as heat and dryness, are carried to the head and cause their most pronounced symptoms there.

In an age before refrigeration, damp foodstuffs were especially prone to spoil. Dampness carried the energies of Yin, which sank in the body through the stomach to the abdomen. The front of the body, that is, the chest and abdomen, came to be recognized as the place where Yin channels flow. These carry Yin energy and have the function of nourishing the body. The most severe symptoms of exposure to damp and cold, such as chest colds and peptic ulcers, are gradually felt where the Yin channels flow.

By the end of the second century B.C., Chinese doctors came to believe that excesses of Yang and Yin could explain all the visible symptoms of disease. An excess of Yang is associated with heat, and an excess of Yin is associated with cold. Therefore an individual experiencing fever is suffering an excess of Yang, and the experience of chill is due to an excess of Yin.

The ancient physicians noticed many other patterns of Yang and Yin. Motion is made possible by Yang. Fidgeting, insomnia, nervousness, and twitching muscles are due to excesses of Yang. Rest is made possible by Yin. Sleepiness and fatigue are signs of an excess of Yin. Overabundance of Yang and Yin were also seen in dryness and dampness, hardness and softness, speed and slowness, and excitement and inhibition, respectively. Diseases caused by excessive Yang came on quickly and struck people who had been in good physical condition. Diseases caused by excessive Yin came on slowly, tended to linger, and tended to strike the chronically disabled and the elderly.

Diagnosis of disease by Yang and Yin in Japan today is a process not fundamentally different from any diagnostic process in Western medicine. Since a diagnosis of Yang or Yin is important to choosing an effective herbal medicine, many Japanese physicians use a checklist similar to the scoring system in Table 2.4.

Table 2.4 Diagnostic Scoring System for Yang and Yin

A score of +7 or more indicates a condition of Yang.
A score of -7 or less indicates a condition of Yin.

Yang Signs	**Point Value**	**Yin Signs**	**Point Value**
Feeling hot at room temperature, desire for thin clothes	+4	Feeling cold at room temperature, desire for heavy clothes	-4
Desire for cold drinks or cold showers	+2	Desire for hot drinks or hot baths	-2
Red face	+2	Pale face	-2
Body temperature over 98.6° F (37° C)	+2	Body temperature under 98.6°F (37° C)	-2
Red tip of the tongue	+2	Coldness of the back or neck	-2
Burning diarrhea	+2	Diarrhea without burning sensation	-2
Burning sensation during urination, strong steam	+2	Weak stream during urination	-2
Pungent fecal odor	+1	Faint fecal odor	-1
Fast pulse	+1	Impaired hearing, difficulties in speaking clearly	-1
Skipped heart beats	+1	Cold hands or feet	-1

Excess and deficiency. Yang and Yin may be too little or too much to perform their normal functions in the body. In Japanese, conditions of excess and deficiency are known as *jitsu* and *kyo*, respectively.

When an organ is *jitsu* or has too much *ki*, it may be overworked. Alternatively, it may have tapped too much of the body's energy, causing an energy blockage and preventing other organs from being adequately nourished with life force. Conditions of excess are most commonly seen in the earliest stages of disease, when the immune system is unimpaired. The body throws energy at the invading pernicious influence and creates a variety of symptoms, described by traditional Chinese herbal physician Kaptchuk as a "cluttered clinical landscape." When *ki* is excessive, disease makes an encounter with a robust life force.

When an organ is *kyo* or has too little *ki*, it is lethargic. It cannot generate or pass on energy to the body as a whole, depriving the body as a whole of its unique contributions to the life force. Deficiency patterns are usually chronic, characteristic of the later stages of disease in which the immune system is too tired to produce symptoms. Dr. Kaptchuk refers to a deficiency state as a "bleak and desolate" clinical landscape.

Excessive *ki* is more likely to be found in a single organ than in the body as a whole. It is likely to result from the body's vigorous immune response to a disease, intended to keep it from spreading to the body. Deficient *ki* is more likely to be found in the body as a whole than in a single organ. It is likely to result from an exhaustion of nutrients by a prolonged immune response.

Japanese physicians also use a simple checklist to diagnose conditions of *ki* excess and deficiency. The scoring chart shown in table 2.5 refers to energy levels in the body as a whole.

Table 2.5 Excess and Deficiency of *Ki*

A score of +6 or more indicates a condition of excess, while a total score of -6 points or less indicates a condition of deficiency. Scores between +6 and -6 describe a status of ki between excess and deficiency.

Symptom	Point Value	Symptom	Point Value
Severe pain in chest or abdomen	+4	Hernia or prolapse	-4
Racing pulse	+4	Sound of fluctuating liquid in the stomach	-4
Eczema, skin pain	+2	Sweating at night	-2
Painful muscle tension	+2	No constipation, no odor of feces	-2
Offensive fecal odor, constipation	+2	Loose skin	-2
"Apple" or "beer belly" obesity	+2	Slow pulse	-2
Abdominal tension	+2	Loose abdominal muscles	-2
Bright eyes, strong voice	+1	Dull eyes, weak voice	-1
Normal skin color	+1	Pale skin	-1
Tight skin	+1	Sweating without physical exertion	-1

Japanese physicians then use the diagnoses of Yang or Yin and excess or deficiency together to prescribe an appropriate herbal formula. The herbs are chosen to decrease energy when *ki* is excessive or increase energy when *ki* is deficient. They are also designed to ensure that neither Yang nor Yin predominates.

An example of how the scoring may be used is that of a 71-year-old man who comes in to see his doctor for treatment of chronic bloating and gas. Bowel movement is painful and passing gas brings no relief. His EKG is satisfactory but shows skipped heartbeats (a Yang sign). His stomach rumbles (a sign of deficient *ki*). Five years earlier he had had surgery for prostate cancer but continued to have urinary difficulties, including a weak stream of urination (Yin sign) and tendency to need to urinate at night. Frequently, since his wife passed away two years ago, he wakes up at night in a cold sweat (Yin sign, sign of deficient *ki*). He catches colds easily, once or twice a month in the winter months, and has cold hands and feet (Yin sign). He keeps his coat on even though the office is well-heated (Yin sign). Ever since his other doctor changed blood-pressure medications, he has a tendency to get dizzy or even pass out when moving from a seated position to a standing position.

Scoring with Tables 2.4 and 2.5 indicates that this 71-year-old man has an excess of Yin with deficient *ki*. The effective herbal treatment for his condition is Minor Construct the Middle Formula, found in table 2.6.

When more than one formula is suggested for a combination of Yang and Yin with excess or deficiency, consideration of specific symptoms leads to the choice of the best formula. Part 2 of this book lists symptom patterns treated by each formula, with explanations of how the formulas treat medically diagnosed diseases.

Table 2.6 Herbal Formulas for Yang and Yin, Excess and Deficiency

Yang Symptoms, Excessive Ki	Cinnamon and Poria Pill (page 237) Goddess Powder (page 166) Ledebouriella Powder that Sagely Unblocks (page 171) Major Bupleurum Formula (page 177) Major Order the Qi Formula (page 265) Minor Bupleurum Formula (page 185) Peach Pit Decoction to Order the Qi (page 269)
Yang Symptoms, Deficient Ki	Aconite (page 104) Bupleurum and Cinnamon Formula (page 222) Calm the Stomach and Poria Powder (page 228) Cinnamon Formula (page 133) Clear Summerheat and Augment the Qi Formula (page 140) Uncaria Powder (page 211)
Yin Symptoms, Excessive Ki	Augmented Rambling Powder (page 119) Bupleurum, Cinnamon , and Ginger Decoction (page 226) Pinellia Draining Formula (page 274) Tonify the Middle and Augment the Qi Formula (page 206)
Yin Symptoms, Deficient Ki	Evodia Formula (page 243) Ginseng Formula (page 254) Minor Construct the Middle Decoction (page 266) Mysterious Decoction (page 268)

Heat and Cold, Exterior and Interior. Excesses and deficiencies of Yang and Yin may also manifest themselves as heat and cold. A local excess of *ki* can cause heat. A local deficiency of *ki* may cause cold. This is not the "pernicious cold" of Zhang Zhong-jing but the physiological cold of everyday experience.

Heat expresses itself *locally* in the body as:

- Dilation of blood vessels in the hands and feet
- Redness in the face
- Heat in the joints and skin
- Burning pain
- Spasmodic pain
- Thirst and desire for cold drinks
- Rapid pulse
- Heartburn
- Bad breath
- Bitter taste in the mouth
- Burning during urination, or
- Tenesmus, a distressing but ineffectual urge to evacuate the rectum or urinary bladder

Cold expresses itself *locally* in the body as:

- Pale complexion
- Subjective sensation of coldness in the joints or skin
- Muscle spasms
- Desire for hot drinks
- Slow pulse
- Coldness in the neck and back
- Cold hands or feet
- Watery diarrhea, or
- Tendency for oozing wounds.

Disturbances of heat and cold may occur in the inner, outer, or middle layers of the body. Disharmony of the exterior layers of the body manifests itself in the skin, hair, and nails, or in the functions of the brain and central nervous system. Exterior energy disturbances usually invoke an acute illness with a sudden onset of strong symptoms, including headache. Exterior conditions are usually related to what Western medicine would consider an infection.

Disharmony of the middle layers of the body manifests itself in the muscles, bones, cartilage, circulatory system, or the reproductive organs. These illnesses usually do not come on suddenly. They induce ongoing, mild symptoms. Disharmony of the inner layers of the body typically affects the endocrine system. These illnesses are chronic conditions that often concern an individual's constitutional tendencies or basic emotional life.

There are no scoring systems for symptoms of heat and cold or exterior and interior, since these disharmonies tend to affect organs individually rather than the body as a whole. However, there are specific herbal remedies for combinations of disharmonies of heat and cold and exterior and interior that are used in Japanese Kampo medicine. Examples of these are shown in Table 2.7.

Table 2.7 Herbal Formulas for Heat and Cold, Exterior and Interior

Localization	Symptom	Formula
Cold, exterior	Sore throat, stiff muscles, runny nose, chills	Ephedra, Asiasarum, and Prepared Aconite Formula (page 242)
Cold, middle	Runny nose, asthma with expectoration of phlegm	Minor Bluegreen Dragon Formula (page 185)
Cold, interior	Abdominal pain, diarrhea, frequent urination	Major Construct the Middle Formula (page 180)
Heat, exterior	Red face, headache, hot flashes	Gypsum and Atractylodis Formula (page 258)
Heat, middle	Bitter, sticky taste in the mouth, "green at the gills" skin coloration	Major Bupleurum Formula (page 177) Japanese Lily Formula (page 262)
Heat, interior	Rapid pulse, thirst, feeling of heat throughout the body, sticky sweat	Ginseng Formula (page 254) White Tiger Formula (page 286)
Subjective sensation of cold, exterior	Chills, headache, tension of shoulder and neck muscles	Ephedra Formula (page 157)

Yang and Yin, excess and deficiency, hot and cold, and interior and exterior are known collectively as the Eight Principle Patterns. East Asian traditional medicine refers to them constantly. In Chinese medicine these eight patterns are termed the *Ba-Gang Bian-Zheng.*

Ba means eight. *Gang* was originally a term for a guide rope for a fishing net. It refers to essentials, parameters, or guiding principles. *Bian-zheng* is a common term in Chinese medical literature. *Bian* means to clarify, while a *zheng* is an ailment. Together the *Ba-Gang Bian-Zheng* are the diagnostic syndromes of traditional Chinese and Japanese Kampo herbal medicine. Yang and Yin are of primary importance because of their breadth of definition, and the other six patterns are ultimately explained in terms of Yang and Yin. Even together with the Six Stages of Disease, however, the Eight Principle Patterns are not enough to describe the body.

The Three Textures of Yang and Yin. The physicians of ancient East Asia sought to subdivide the energy body further into three textures, *ki,* blood, and fluids. Traditional Chinese medicine developed a special category of fluids known as phlegm, which may be either substantial (a discharge, such as mucus) or non-substantial (a stagnant emotion). Phlegm can build up so that the activities modern medicine associates with the central nervous system are impeded. A facial tic or twitch, for instance, might be described and treated as a manifestation of phlegm. Together, the three textures are extraordinarily useful in describing the disease process of either Yang or Yin.

Ki is a far more ancient concept than Yang and Yin. More than 5,000 years ago, physicians in India and China came to understand that all things in the universe relate to each other. There is a oneness and wholeness that pervades the entirety of existence, and, energetically, everything is connected as one body.

Ki is the capacity of any part of the universe to relate to the whole. It requires energy, but is not energy. It is the catalyst for relationship and interrelationship.

In the human body, *ki* is evidenced by the ability of one part of the body to relate other parts of the body, or to relate food or energy to the body through its normal functions. *Ki* may be deficient or excessive. For instance, if the digestive system lacks *ki*, it cannot relate food to the body. The result is diarrhea. If the circulatory system lacks *ki*, the blood vessels cannot relate blood to its proper channels. The result may be bleeding or bruising. If the "hollow organs" lack *ki*, they may not be able to hold their shape. The result may be hernia or prolapse. Excessive *ki* causes an organ to generate energy it cannot use. The result is heat, which causes fever.

Ki powers both Yang and Yin. In extreme cases, *ki* can become so deficient it depletes either Yang or Yin. When Yang collapses from deficient *ki*, the result is cold. Its manifestations are chills and external tissues that are cold to the touch. When Yin collapses from deficient *ki*, the result is "fire." Its manifestations are abundant perspiration, released by tissues that can no longer hold fluids, and external tissues that can no longer hold heat and are hot to the touch.

Ki deficiency is one of the most common diagnoses of modern Kampo medicine. Kampo medicine has a theory of deficient energy due to genetic causes, but more often than not, the root of *ki* deficiency is thought to be insufficient intake of energy from the air, that is, improper breathing. *Ki* deficiency also may stem from malnutrition, or from dissipation of energy from the "kidneys" by excessive sexual activity, excessive consumption of sugars, or hormonal imbalances.

The symptoms of deficient *ki* are intuitive:

- Physical weakness or fatigue.
- Depression or declining intellectual capacity.
- Declining sexual desire, erectile dysfunction.
- Prolapse of interior organs (uterus, rectum).
- Symptoms of declining nerve activity or insufficient circulation.
- Declining activity in life as a whole.

The most obvious symptom of a deficiency of *ki* is fatigue. The root cause of this deficiency is usually nutritional, and the Kampo approach to nutritional deficiency illustrates an important conceptual difference between East Asian and Western medicine.

A deficiency of nutritional *ki* clearly relates to a failure to consume adequate nourishment. In times of abundance, this can only be due to loss of appetite. Physicians trained in Kampo look for teeth marks to confirm "eating one's own tongue" as sign of loss of appetite. An absence of *ki* in the digestive system leads to a slightly uncomfortable feeling after eating a full meal. As a result, the patient constantly nibbles and snacks and picks at food, consuming more and more calories with less and less nourishment. The body is deprived of the full measure of *ki* a balanced meal provides, so the muscles become weak and there is constant fatigue. On the other hand, *loss* of appetite has led to excessive consumption of food and there is weight gain.

The Kampo treatment of the deficiency of nutritional *ki* is similarly counterintuitive to those of us grounded in Western nutritional concepts. To counteract hunger, patients (including patients with controlled diabetes) are encouraged to eat *measured* amounts of sugar, typically included in the prescribed formula with herbs. Sugar does more than provide a quick energy boost. It changes the fluid balance of the digestive tract so that it is "moistened." This relieves discomfort after eating a full meal, which in turn encourages consumption of normal nutrition. Sugar is antitussive, that is, it helps stop chronic coughing and restores the nutritional *ki* of the lungs. It helps prevent colds and, in East Asian thought, helps shy people find the courage to act boldly.

A similar effect is found in another commonly prescribed carbohydrate, rice. It is critical to note that Kampo medicine uses these carbohydrates as medicines to restore deficient *ki* only in measured amounts. It is also important to note that sugar and rice are only two of many remedies for deficient *ki*.

Ginseng intensifies existing *ki* and stimulates the production of body fluids, both those that regulate digestion and the "fluids" that correspond to hormones. Astragalus intensifies *ki* and stimulates the immune system in the First, Second, and Third Stages of Disease. White actractylodis acts as tonic to the digestive system and a diuretic, and also intensifies *ki*. Poria (hoelen) mushroom harmonizes the energies of the digestive system, removes water weight, and acts as a sedative. Licorice is antitoxic, lowers fevers, stops dry cough, and also intensifies existing *ki*.

Physicians in Japan often diagnose deficient *ki* with a checklist like that shown in Table 2.8. Diagnosis of some categories, such as lack of will power, is entirely subjective. Diagnosis in other categories is sufficiently commonsensical that even persons without formal training in Kampo can recognize symptoms with confidence.

Table 2.8 Diagnostic Scoring System for *Ki* Deficiency

A score of 15 points or more indicates ki deficiency.

Symptom	Points	Symptom	Points
Collapsed organs (weak bladder, hemorrhoids, hernia, prolapsed uterus)	5	Lack of willpower	5
Easy fatigue after exercise	5	General fatigue, sensitivity to cold	5
Daytime sleepiness	2	Swelling, water retention, or sweaty palms or feet	2
Frequent infection	2	Slow pulse without athletic training	2
"Jelly belly," or reduced tension in lower abdomen	2	"Flabby" muscles	3
Feeble voice	3	Loss of appetite	2
Frequent diarrhea	2	Easily frightened	2

Using the diagnostic score as a key to an appropriate diagnosis, it is then possible to lock in an herbal formula that will improve symptoms. The primary "energizing" herbs of Oriental medicine are cinnamon and ginseng. Cinnamon "wakes up" the *ki*, causing it to flow upward in the body. Ginseng intensifies energy and also increases the production of fluids. The ancient Kampo formulas combined these key herbs with others to lock in a needed effect, as shown in table 2.9.

Table 2.9 Herbal Remedies for Deficient *Ki*

Remedies	Possible Symptoms	Formula
Remedies Containing Cinnamon	Eczema, inflammation anywhere in the body, easy fatigue, pain around the navel (in women and children) lack of bladder control, (in men) impotence, nervousness, nightmares	Astragalus Formula (page 116) Cinnamon, Dragon Bone, and Oyster Shell Formula (page 137)
	Bleeding hemorrhoids, herpes outbreaks, cold-naturedness, chronic and mild abdominal pain	Dong Quai Rejuvenation Formula (page 241)
	Age spots or freckles, hot hands or feet, pain around the navel, difficulty controlling urination	Minor Construct the Middle Formula (page 266)
Remedies Containing Ginseng	Summertime fatigue, especially with loss of weight during summer, occasional diarrhea or fever.	Clear Summerheat and Augment the Qi Formula (page 140)
	Headache, vomiting, diarrhea, rumbling stomach, tender feeling above stomach, difficulty keeping warm	Evodia Formula (page 243)
	Loss of appetite, bloating, gas	Four-Gentlemen Formula (page 251)
	Dizziness, headaches, sensitivity to cold, common cold, tired after eating	Uncaria Powder (page 211)
	Diarrhea, heartburn, chronic mild chest pain	Ginseng Formula (page 254)
	Loss of appetite, nausea, vomiting, stomach rumbles	Six-Gentlemen Formula (page 280)
	Loss of appetite, general fatigue, mild fever	Tonify the Middle and Augment the *Qi* Formula (page 206)

Ki deficiency is a frequent cause of chronic health conditions in children who are otherwise generally healthy. Dr. Katsutoshi Terasawa of Toyama Medical and Pharmaceutical University recounts the examination of an eight-year-old girl who wet her bed two or three times a night. Constantly having to get up at night, she was fatigued and sleepy during the day (4 points of the *ki* Deficiency Scale). She also had sweaty palms (4 points), was sensitive to cold (5 points), and tired easily while playing (5 points). Her *ki* deficiency score of 19 indicated a need for "energizing" herbs.

Dr. Terasawa gave the girl Astragalus Formula for two weeks. This reduced her nighttime urination, but did not completely eliminate it. Dr. Terasawa added Cinnamon, Dragon Bone, and Oyster Shell Formula to her treatment. Her feeling of fatigue completely disappeared, and she only had to get up to go to the bathroom once per night.

Even when *ki* is not deficient, it may be depressed. This is a condition in which the energy of relationship does not circulate throughout the body. While the energy is adequate for the body's needs, it is static in a single organ. It can cause a feeling of heaving, constriction, or strangulation, and even transform itself into lumps, swelling, hardness, or stiffness.

The oldest teachings of Japanese Traditional Medicine identify different symptoms of blocked *ki* in the Five Rings of the Body. In traditional Japanese medicine, the strength of the outward or Yang body was to reside in five circular body parts. These were the elbows, knees, and head. In the inner, Yin body, there are also five rings at the same points. The knees are referred to as the Ring of Earth, the navel is referred to as the Ring of Water, the chest is referred to as the Ring of Fire, the face is referred to as the Ring of Wind, and the top of the head is referred to as the Ring of *Ku* (not *ki*), or the ring of the "eternal void."

Static or depressed *ki* in the Ring of *Ku*, in the head, can cause depression, attention deficit, or just a heavy feeling in the head. Static or depressed *ki* in the Ring of Wind, in the face, can cause a feeling of stiffness, swelling, or numbness. Static or depressed *ki* between the Ring of *Ku* and the Ring of Water, in the throat, can cause a feeling of constriction and strangulation. This is a sensation of having a lump in the throat. Static or depressed *ki* in the Ring of Fire itself, over the heart or in the chest, can cause a feeling of distress, accumulation of fluids in the chest, and difficulty breathing. Stasis of *ki* on the sides of the chest results in tenderness, pain, and pressure. *Ki* blockage at the Ring of Water, or abdomen, results in gas and flatulence. Static or depressed *ki* in any of the five circular things could cause swelling, hardening, stiffness, or a loss of sensation. Static or depressed *ki* of *ku* leads to unpredictable periods of colic-like pain, ongoing dull pain, self-pity, and constant complaining about one's condition, or hypochondria.

Ki depression or blockage nearly always causes chronic disease. Kampo medicine associates *ki* blockage with chronic middle ear infections and asthma. Interestingly, modern medicine associates chronic middle ear infections and asthma with accumulations of immune cells known as eosinophils. Chronic ear infections in particular produce discharges that are more viscous, thicker, and darker, and cause the mucous membranes of the ear to become thickened with an excess of these immune cells. This medically identifiable immune-system blockage corresponds to the *ki* blockage described in Kampo.

The understanding of static and depressed vital energies in traditional Japanese medicine roughly corresponds to its Chinese counterpart. Japanese physicians frequently use a checklist to diagnose a condition of depressed *ki* from its symptoms, as shown in table 2.10.

Table 2.10. Diagnosis of Depressed or Static *Ki.*

A score of 15 or more indicates depressed ki.

Symptom	Points	Symptom	Points
Depression	9	Lump in the throat	6
Difficulty getting up in the morning	4	Chest cold, or stuffy chest, asthma, or emphysema	4
Heavy feeling in the head, as if wearing a hat	4	Pain or heaviness in the sides of the chest.	4
Bloating, gas	4	Pain that seems to drift through the body	4
Stomach rumbles	4	Frequent flatulence	3
Feeling of incomplete urination	2	Hiccups	2

Kampo treats the symptoms of depressed *ki* with two basic formulas. One of them, Cyperus and Perilla Formula (discussed in more detail on page 234), is composed for five herbs: cyperus rhizome, perilla leaf, bitter orange peel, ginger, and licorice. The other, Pinellia and Magnolia Bark Formula (page 272) also contains five herbs: magnolia bark, pinellia root, perilla leaf, poria mushroom, and ginger.

Cyperus and pinellia are the primary "unblocking" herbs in Kampo medicine. In terms of traditional medicine, cyperus is particularly useful for releasing emotional "blockages," associated energetically with the liver. Pinellia stops vomiting and releases fluid "blockages" by eliminating excessive body fluid. Whole bitter orange stimulates the flow of energy below the ribcage. Bitter orange peel stimulates the flow of *ki* throughout the body and helps eliminate moisture in the form water retention, incomplete urination, or swelling. Bupleurum fortifies cyperus in releasing emotional blockages and also lowers fevers. Magnolia bark balances energy flows throughout the body, removes bloat and gas, and eliminates excessive body fluids. Perilla leaf regulates digestion and stops sweating. These herbs are used in the formulas detailed in table 2.11.

Table 2.11. Modifications of Basic Formulas to Treat Depressed *Ki*.

Formulas Containing	Possible Symptoms	Combination of Herbs
Cyperus and Perilla Formula	Sluggish digestion, loss of appetite, restlessness, headache, stuffy nose	Cyperus and Perilla Formula (page 239)
	Hot flashes, back pain, cold feet, insomnia, heavy feeling in the head like wearing a cap or hat	Goddess Powder (page 166)
Magnolia and Pinellia Formula	Lump in the throat, bloat, sluggish digestion, plus bitter taste in the mouth, mild fever	Bupleurum and Magnolia Formula (page 122)
	Lump in the throat, bloat, sluggish digestion	Pinellia and Magnolia Bark Formula (page 272)

The problem of deficient *ki* was a principal concern of the *Yellow Emperor's Classic of Internal Medicine.* The physicians attending the Yellow Emperor believed that this kind of energy problem was due to either excessive thinking or excessive emotional strain. They maintained that the single most important measure one can to take to prevent both the physical symptoms of depressed *ki* and other kinds of emotional problems is to avoid excessive mental work. The very first chapter *Simple Questions* asked by the Yellow Emperor states, "One should live a quiet life with few desires so that one can preserve one's *ki* and guard one's mind is order to avoid disease. If emotions are absent and craving is curbed, the heart is peaceful and there is no fear."

Thus, in order to guard one's mind, the ancient Taoist sages counseled the Yellow Emperor to avoid excessive thinking, avoid excessive craving, and avoid distracting thoughts. Mimicking the combinations of five herbs in the formula Cypress and Perilla Powder for depressed *ki,* they formulated a "prescription" of their own:

- Not thinking too much (nourishes the heart)
- Restraining anger (nourishes the emotional reserves)
- Restraining sexual desires (preserves the genetic inheritance)
- Careful talking (saves breath)
- Regulating diet (stimulates the nutritive *ki*)

Even when *ki* is neither deficient nor in excess, it may be rebellious, refusing to flow in its normal directions. For instance, the stomach normally relates food to organs below it, that is, it sends digested food to the intestine. When stomach *ki* rebels, it flows in the opposite of its intended direction. Rebellious *ki* of the stomach causes belching, hiccups, nausea, and vomiting.

Whereas Traditional Chinese Medicine speaks of rebellious *ki,* modern Japanese herbal practice typically refers to "*ki* imbalance." This condition results from *ki*'s failure to circulate between the inner and outer layers of the body, or between the upper and lower parts of the body.

When *ki* is out of balance at the level of the abdomen, there is a feeling of distress and tightness moving upwards to the chest. There is usually also a loss of control of the *hara*, that is, a loss of psychic harmony. When *ki* is out of balance at the chest, there is a feeling of fullness in the chest accompanied by coughing. There may be a lump in the throat, or impatience, aggressiveness, and irritability. When *ki* is out of balance just above the stomach, there is mild nausea and burping up of gastric juices. And *ki* out of balance at any of the four extremities (the hands and feet) causes coldness and pain that moves up to the head and brain, as well as symptoms that might otherwise be considered a severe *ki* deficiency.

Table 2.12. Diagnostic Checklist for *Ki* Imbalance

A score of 15 or more indicates *ki* imbalance.

Symptom	Points	Symptom	Points
Abdominal palpitations	7	Feeling hot in the upper part of the body, cold in the lower part of the body	7
Coughing attacks, irritability	5	Red face	5
Racing heart for no apparent reason	4	Impatience	4
Vomiting	4	Recurrent headaches	4
Painful spasms in the abdomen	3	Easily frightened	3
Cold hands and feet	2	Sweaty hands and feet	2

Most of the formulas for *ki* imbalance contain cinnamon bark and licorice. Cinnamon stimulates the flow of energy throughout the body, while licorice calms upset stomach. Other herbs added to these two include coptis to stop stomach palpitations, cyperus to relieve pain and prevent infection, evodia to "heat up" cold symptoms, pinellia for a feeling of stuffed stomach, perilla to stimulate energy circulation, and schisandra to stop cough. Other formulas that do not contain cinnamon and licorice are used for specialized combinations of symptoms.

Table 2.13. Formulas to Treat Imbalances of *Ki*.

Herbs	Symptoms	Combination of Herbs
Formulas Containing Cinnamon and Licorice	Abdominal palpitations, fearfulness, insomnia, fidgeting	Cinnamon, Dragon Bone, and Oyster Shell Formula (page 137)
	Nausea, vomiting, stomach pain, feeling of heat in the upper part of the body and cold in the lower part of the body	Coptis Formula (page 238)
	Feeling of heat in the upper part of the body and cold in the lower part of the body, constipation, anxiety, restlessness.	Peach Pit Decoction to Order the *Qi* (page 268)
Other Formulas	Hot flashes, fearfulness, fidgeting	Augmented Rambling Powder (page 119)
	Headache, stomachache, sloshing sounds in the stomach	Evodia Formula (page 243)

Imbalances of *ki* are also typical in people who have what Western medicine would call "psychosomatic" disorders. An example would be a phobia resulting in a panic attack. Dizziness and vertigo, a racing heart, breaking out in a cold sweat, and a mild flushing of the face would be treated with Cinnamon, Dragon Bone, and Oyster Shell Formula (page 137).

Imbalances of *ki* are also typical in people who have peptic ulcers. A common combination of symptoms would be to have a weakness of the digestive system with a feeling of heat in the upper part of the body and cold in the lower part (for example, cold feet). There typically is also a tendency to get colds, hay fever, and an annual case of the flu. This imbalance leaves the sufferer chronically feelings nervous, blushing in social situations, and ill at ease.

Ki out of balance at the level of the stomach frequently presents itself as severe indigestion. Some people will react violently to foods containing gluten, while other people will be unable to tolerate milk. If these symptoms coincide with cold sweat and cold feet, treating the imbalance at this level will help.

Whiplash victims suffer imbalances of *ki* at the level of the abdomen. Even years after the accident, there may be persistent dull pain aggravated by changing weather, or stabbing pains that seem to drift around the neck and back accompanied by sharp headaches. These are due to imbalances of *ki*. The same formulas that relieve imbalances of *ki* causing chronic bloating, water retention, or gas are helpful in treating whiplash.

Blood is impelled by *ki* to flow throughout the body. *Ki* also enables blood to stay within the blood vessels, properly relating to the organs and tissues it serves. The concept of blood in Kampo medicine encompasses blood as it is understood in Western languages and Western medicine, but also includes any transformation of constructive energies that are sent throughout the body.

Blood may be deficient or stagnant, the later condition being the peculiar manifestation of the Third Stage of Disease known as *oketsu*. Blood is a Yin substance. Yin is the energy of containment. When there is not enough blood in circulation, the organs may not have the means to hold their normal energies. Kampo medicine teaches that the loss of blood during menstruation, for example, causes the energy of the liver to lose its ability to hold emotional energy. This leads to the depression and emotional lability of premenstrual syndrome.

Deficient blood may also be the result of inadequate nutrition or loss of blood through injury or disease. Deficient blood fails to carry Yin to the organs. Lacking Yin, the organs cannot hold energies or form. Muscles nourished by deficient blood cannot hold still, and the energies of a liver supplied with deficient blood cannot hold back anger.

In modern terms, the causes of deficient blood may be anemia, wasting diseases, cancer, surgery, hemorrhage of the digestive tract, heavy menstrual periods, bleeding hemorrhoids, drugs, poisons, or exposure to radioactive material, among many others. The results of deficient blood may be loss of weight or muscle mass, pallor, visual disturbances, baldness, wrinkles, cramps, convulsions, and abnormal sensations in the hands and feet, also among many others. The diseases associated with an energy diagnosis of deficient blood include rheumatoid arthritis, collagen diseases, diabetic neuropathy, dermatitis, eczema, pruritus in the elderly, dysmenorrhea, peptic ulcers, bleeding ulcers, Crohn's diseases, and thrombocytopenia. Japanese doctors make a diagnosis of blood deficiency on symptoms summarized in table 2.14. (Formulas to treat deficient blood syndromes are discussed in Part 2.)

Table 2.14. Diagnostic Checklist for Deficient Blood

A score of 15 points or more indicates deficient blood.

Symptom	Points	Symptom	Points
Dry, rough skin	7	Eyestrain	6
Muscle cramps	5	Pale complexion	5
Dizziness	4	Broken nails	4
Hair loss	4	Muscular weakness	3
Insomnia	3	Loss of tactile sensation in the skin	3
Scanty or missed menstrual periods	3	Tension in the abdominal muscles	3

Oketsu, or stagnant blood, occurs when blood is unable to flow smoothly. It results in localized pain, which worsens with pressure. Over time, stagnant blood solidifies to cause swellings, cysts, and tumors.

Blood may also be "hot." In the terminology of traditional East Asian medicine, hot blood is due to exposure to external wind. In the Japanese tradition, wind captures the energy of diversity. The diseases of the wind are the diseases of diversity. Some of these diseases obviously "come in on a wind," such as colds, flu, allergy, and tension-related "pain in the neck." When these conditions make the blood hot, they cause itching, heat, redness, and outbreaks on the skin.

Table 2.15 Scoring System for *Oketsu* Syndrome.

A score of 8 points or more indicates a mild blood stasis and a score of 16 points or more indicates a severe blood stasis.

Symptom	Points	
	Men	Women
Dark circles under the eyes	4	4
Red gums	4	2
Red tongue	4	4
Hemorrhoids	4	2
Tenderness on the left side of the navel	4	4
"Spider" veins	2	2
Dysmennorhea	2	4
Tenderness on the right side of the navel	2	2
Tenderness on the sides below the rib cage	2	2
Tenderness over the lower abdomen	2	2
Facial freckles	1	1
Rough skin	1	2
Red lips	1	1
Rash on the palms	1	2

No diagnostic category of traditional Japanese medicine has been subjected to greater scientific scrutiny than *oketsu*. Scientific research led by Dr. Nobuyoshi Hagino at the University of Texas at San Antonio has found that in *oketsu* the cells composing the delicate linings of veins, arteries, and capillaries become "tired." There is a deficiency of positively charged potassium ions in the extracellular space, which leads to a smaller charge across the membrane of the cells. These run-down cells cannot generate a charge to attract glucose and other nutrients, and they cannot discharge toxic amounts of calcium. They become inefficient and eventually die. The herbs used in Kampo formulas release potassium and "recharge" tired cells.

Table 2.16 Formulas to Treat *Oketsu*

Energy Status	Accompanying Symptoms	Corresponding Formula
Excessive *ki*	Hardness or resistance to pressure around the navel	Rhubarb and Moutan Formula (page 279)
	Abdominal tenderness, unbalanced distribution of *ki*	Peach Pit Decoction to Order the Qi (page 269)
Ki neither excessive nor deficient	Tenderness on the right side under the ribs, fearfulness	Augmented Rambling Powder (page 119)
	Joint pain, neuralgia, loss of sensation, deficiency of blood	Relax the Channels and Invigorate the Blood Formula (page 191)
Deficient *ki*	Anemia, hemorrhage (with symptoms of blood stasis)	Dong Quai and Peony Formula (page 150)

Fluids. Just as the blood is a condensed form of *ki* that the body makes from food, the fluids are a condensed form of *ki* that the body makes from blood. Yang fluids are clear and move upward in the body with the energies of the immune system. They provide tears, sweat, saliva, and mucus. Yin fluids are colored and move downward in the body. These fluids lubricate the joints with synovial fluid, nourish the brain and spinal cord with cerebrospinal fluid, and enable the function of the sensory organs—the eyes, ears, nose, and mouth.

Deficient fluids are usually caused by prolonged loss of fluids through sweating, diarrhea, or vomiting. Deficient fluids affect the joints and the sense organs. Excess fluids are usually associated with deficient energy in:

- The lungs, leading to fluid accumulations in the body, face, and hands, or
- The "spleen" (digestive system), leading to fluid accumulations in the abdomen, or
- The kidneys, leading to fluid accumulations in the legs and ankles.

Fluids are constantly formed and constantly eliminated by the body. The lungs disperse them upward and the kidneys disperse them downward. When a failure of these organs allows them to accumulate, the result is phlegm.

Phlegm may be substantial or non-substantial. The ancient texts describe substantial phlegm as "having a form." This is the thick mucus that accumulates during bronchial infections and other lung diseases. As lung disease progresses, substantial phlegm changes color. It is first clear, then yellow, then green, and finally reddish-brown.

The ancient texts describe non-substantial phlegm as "having no form." It accumulates in the joints, causing bone deformations, or causes lumps or cysts. In chronic diseases traditional East Asian medicine associates with the kidneys, such as diabetes or adrenal disease, phlegm frequently clogs the channels through which *ki* circulates through the body. This causes twitches, shaking, and mood swings.

Unlike the other branches of traditional East Asian herbal medicine, Japanese Kampo does not make fine distinctions between the various types of fluids. In Kampo, blood is a liquid that is red and fluids are liquids that are not. There may be an imbalance of secretion, as in excessive urination, watery diarrhea, drooling, or runny nose, or there may be "fluid stasis," as in edema, ascites, and sloshing fluids in the digestive tract. These fluid imbalances are perceived by the patient as swollen joints (especially in the morning), a feeling of heaviness throughout the body, palpitations, motion sickness, tinnitus, headache, nausea, vomiting, diarrhea, or thirst.

Stasis of fluids may affect the entire body, as in diarrhea, dizziness, and anasarca (a generalized accumulation of serum in the connective tissue). This condition may be limited to the outer layers of the body, skin and joints, when there is edema, swelling of joints, or swelling and stiffness of joints in the morning. It may be limited to the chest, causing respiratory distress and a feeling of accumulated fluids in the chest, coughing with phlegm, racing pulse, or accumulation of fluids in the chest during congestive heart failure. And stasis of fluids may be epigastric, causing "stomach rumbles," nausea, vomiting, and diarrhea.

Sometimes the diagnosis of static fluids is very easy to make. Congestive heart failure, ascites, and in general any tendency for swelling always indicate static fluids. Other symptoms are noted in the checklist in table 2.17.

Table 2.17. Diagnostic Scoring System for Stasis of Fluids.

A total score of 13 points or more indicates stasis of body fluids.

Symptom	Points	Symptom	Points
Any edema	15	Congestive heart failure, ascites, fluid in the lungs or around the heart	15
Excessive urination	7	Stiff joints in the morning	7
Dizziness	5	Passing out when rising from seated position	5
Motion sickness	5	Watery diarrhea	5
Palpitations above the umbilicus	5	Frequent urination	5
Throbbing headache	4	Foamy saliva	4
Nausea, vomiting	3	Feeling of heaviness throughout the body	3
Runny nose	3	Drooling	3

Health conditions involving static fluids are among those most helped by Kampo. For this reason, Japanese herbal medicine has a considerable repertoire of formulas to "move water" into its natural channels in the body. Most of the formulas contain atractylodis and poria to "break the dam" holding back normal fluid circulation, and cinnamon and licorice to restore the normal circulation of *ki*.

Although the scientific understanding of how these formulas work is in its infancy, preliminary results of laboratory tests in Japan find that certain herbs in the formulas modify local immune responses in tissues. Changing the speed of the immune process, these herbs stop inflammation and restore circulation. Other herbs act directly but gently on the circulatory system to speed the removal of fluids from swollen tissues.

Formulas to relieve static fluids affecting the entire body are listed in table 2.18, in the skin, table 2.19, the chest, table 2.20, and in the epigastric area, table 2.21.

Table 2.18. Formulas for Stasis of Fluids Affecting the Entire Body

Energy Status	Accompanying Symptoms	Corresponding Formula
Excessive *Ki*	Painful urination, fearfulness, excessive urination, pelvic inflammation, genital discharge	Dong Quai and Gentian Formula (page 147)
	Abdominal distention, constipation, swollen and/or stiff joints in the morning	Ledebouriella Powder that Sagely Unblocks (page 171)
Ki neither excessive nor deficient	Loss of appetite, swelling, thirst	Bupleurum and Poria Formula (page 126)
	Scanty urination, tendency to perspire easily, thirst, vomiting, headache, diarrhea, sound of fluctuation liquid in the stomach	Five-Ingredient Powder with Poria (page 248)
	Scanty urination, painful urination, thirst, lack of natural perspiration	Polyporus Formula (page 188)
Deficient *Ki*	Easy fatigue, muscle pain, morning stiffness, scanty urination, swelling	Aconite Formula (page 104)
	Anemia, scanty or missed menstrual periods, cold hands and feet, swelling, abdominal pain, sound of fluctuating liquid in the stomach	Dong Quai and Peony Formula (page 150)
	Easy fatigue, failure to urinate, tendency for swelling, cold feet, prostate enlargement	Eight-Ingredient Pill Rehmannia (page 153)
	Easy fatigue, vertigo, edema, scanty urination, diarrhea, feeling of cold throughout the body	True Warrior Decoction (page 208)

Table 2.19. Formulas for Stasis of Fluids Affecting the Skin

Energy Status	Accompanying Symptoms	Corresponding Formula
Ki neither excessive nor deficient	Facial swelling, scanty urination, thirst, joint pain	Gypsum and Atractylodis Formula (page 258)
Deficient Ki	Anemia, edema, easy fatigue, reduced muscle power of the legs	Great Ledebouriella Formula (page 255)
	Obesity, swelling, scanty urination, absence of thirst, feeling of heaviness in the whole body	Stephania and Astragalus Formula (page 197)

Table 2.20. Formulas for Stasis of Fluids Affecting the Chest

Energy Status	Accompanying Symptoms	Corresponding Formula
Ki neither excessive nor deficient	Asthma, cough, chest pain, bitter taste in the mouth, nausea, mild fever	Mysterious Decoction (page 268)
Deficient *Ki*	Asthma, cough, runny nose, watery sputum, sound of fluctuating liquid in the stomach, excessive perspiration	Minor Bluegreen Dragon Decoction (page 182)

Table 2.21. Formulas for Stasis of Fluids Affecting the Epigastric Region

Energy Status	Accompanying Symptoms	Corresponding Formula
Ki neither excessive nor deficient	Dry mouth, failure to take fluids, jaundice, loss of appetite, abdominal swelling, stomach rumbles, headache, dizziness	Artemisia Formula (page 219)
Deficient *Ki*	Food poisoning, diarrhea, scanty urination	Calm the Stomach and Poria Formula (page 228)
	Chronic diarrhea	Cinnamon Formula (page 133)
	Cold hands and feet, headache, vomiting	Evodia Formula (page 243)
	Headache, intolerance of low room temperatures, easy fatigue, stuffy feeling in the head, sound of fluctuating liquid in the stomach	Uncaria Powder (page 211)
	Sound of fluctuating liquid in the stomach, nausea, vomiting, headache, racing pulse	Two-Cured Formula (page 282)

The Six Stages of Disease, the Eight Diagnostic Principles, and the Three Fluids all contribute to Kampo's understanding of disease. The understanding of the human capacity to relate the energies of health and disease to the greater universe, however, requires an understanding of the five organs: the heart, lungs, liver, stomach, and kidneys. These are the Five Faces of Yang and Yin.

Chapter 3:

The Five Faces of Yang and Yin

The most spectacular advance in the field of medicine of the early twenty-first century A.D. heralded in the summer of 2000 by the mass media is the coding of the human genome. The diagnostic tools of the twentieth century brought a revolution in health care, but they were premised on the a concept similar to "one size fits all." That is, blood tests, CAT scans, X rays, and other technological tools basically compare a sick patient to expectations. Deviation from the norm is the measure of disease. What is needed is a comprehensive way to relate symptoms of disease to their genetic causes, so that illness can be prevented.

The new "map" of the human genome represents a giant leap forward in the tools of medical diagnosis that will allow us to describe the health of individuals at the molecular level. It will no longer be necessary to wait for the symptoms of disease before beginning treatment. It will enable the development of new drugs for previously untreatable diseases, drugs tailored for individuals with far fewer side effects, and the ability to replace faulty genes, and short-circuiting diseases at their source within the patient.

The most spectacular advance in the field of medicine in the early third century B.C. was the theory of the Five Elements. The diagnostic tools of the fourth century B.C. had brought medicine out of the realm of magic, but they too were premised on a concept similar to "one size fits all." The tools of East Asian healing could only discern the energies of Yang and Yin, blood, *ki*, and water when they were in disharmony within the patient. They could not be observed at all until the patient had become sick. What was needed was a comprehensive way to relate these energies that were modified by the experiences of individuals with the world as a whole, so that health could be maintained.

This giant leap forward in the tools of medical diagnosis described the health of individuals at the cosmic level. It was no longer necessary to consider pathogenic energies and the reactions of the body to them. It was now possible to consider the vital energy of life in terms of the functions of human beings in their world. This empowered the development of new drugs for previously untreatable diseases, drugs tailored to individuals, with far fewer side effects, and with the ability to replace faulty energies—short-circuiting diseases at their source within the universe. This discovery was heralded sometime around 300 B.C. by the arrival of giant ants and earthworms.

In the twenty-first century, scientific progress is derived from controlled observations in a laboratory. In the fourth century B.C., intellectual progress was derived from observing the emissary of the divine on earth, the Emperor. About four hundred years after the writing of the *I Ching*, the philosopher Zou Yan said, "Whenever some new dynasty is going to arise, heaven exhibits auspicious signs to the people. During the rise of the Yellow Emperor, large earthworms and large ants appeared. The Emperor said, 'This indicates that earth is in the ascendant, so our color must be yellow, and our affairs must be placed under the sign of earth.' During the rise of Yu the Great, heaven produced plants and trees that did not wither in autumn and winter. The new Emperor said, 'This indicates that Element Wood is in the ascendant, so our color must be green, and our affairs must be placed under the signs of Wood.' "

Through the reigns of five emperors, the sages noted five different types of auspicious signs: Earth, Water, Wood, Fire and Metal. From their observations of those they believed to be heaven's representatives, they concluded that every material thing could be fit into one of these Five Elements. And if every material thing could be categorized in this way, the categories must also apply to the human body.

On a philosophical level, the Five Elements are only measures of harmony. They are transformations, or rings of coincidence. But the sages of the third century B.C. realized that these elements, if they could find them in human beings, would be "resonances" on the same frequency between a part of the body and an event in the outside world.

Physicians looked beyond the Emperor and to their actual experience with patients for the answer. They noticed, for instance, that diseases of the liver were more common in the springtime. The spring was a time in which Wood burst into life, and the liver, which was thought to be associated with Wood, released an outpouring of emotional energy when it was diseased. The color of the face during liver disease is often greenish, which is the color of Wood and the color of spring. The burst of energy of spring corresponded to a burst of energy from a diseased liver, so ancient healers came to expect a burst of energy in the form of anger to accompany liver diseases. The most ancient teachers of Kampo also noticed that, at least in Asia, the most frequent direction of the wind in spring was from the east. An easterly wind seemed to aggravate "liver" diseases, such as headaches and eye pains associated with a sudden burst of emotion or long-standing emotional tension. They noted that the sour taste of pickled foods, which were the last of the previous year's harvest available in the springtime, aggravated the liver. They noted that the predominant sound associated with disturbances of the liver was shouting in anger.

The ancient sages similarly linked the heart with Fire, the lungs with Metal, the digestive organ they called the "spleen" with the Earth, and the kidneys with Water. Their correspondences with the greater world are listed in table 3.1. The sages had identified the Five Faces of Yang and Yin.

Table 3.1. Some of the Correspondences of the Five Elements

	wood	fire	earth	metal	water
Yang Organ	Gallbladder	Small intestine	Stomach	Large intestines	Bladder
Yin Organ	Liver	Heart	Spleen	Lungs	Kidneys
Color	Green	Red	Yellow	White	Black
Direction	East	South	Center	West	North
Emotions	Anger	Joy	Meditation	Sadness	Fear
Planet	Jupiter	Mars	Saturn	Venus	Mercury
Seasons	Spring	Summer	All	Autumn	Winter
Sense Organ	Eyes	Tongue	Mouth	Nose	Ears
Sounds	Shouting	Laughing	Singing	Crying	Groaning
Taste	Sour	Bitter	Sweet	Pungent	Salty
Tissues	Sinews	Vessels	Muscles	Skin	Bones
Weather	Wind	Heart	Dampness	Dryness	Cold

Unfortunately, the neat correspondences of theory did not prove true in actual practice. It was not possible to use one symptom to predict all the others for the element. Medicine needed a less ambitious system of coincidences for clinical use.

In the line of thought that became Japanese herbal medicine, this refinement was not especially complicated. The human body received the Five Elements through five containing, or Yin, organs. These organs received energies from the greater universe. Each was paired with a Yang organ through which the human body sent energy to the greater universe. However, since a deficiency in one organ automatically led to an excess in its paired organ, and vice versa, understanding the five Yin organs is enough to define a system of herbal treatments.

The *liver* exists to ensure the smooth flow of *ki*. It stores blood and regulates the volume of blood in the body as a whole at any given time. The liver stores and releases blood in relation to menstruation in women of reproductive age and in relation to physical activity in all people. When the blood flows to the appropriate places in the body at the appropriate times, tissues are nourished. *The Yellow Emperor's Canon of Internal Medicine* says "When the liver has enough blood, the feet can walk, the hands hold, and the fingers can grasp." The energies of the liver are essential to the functioning of sinews and manifest themselves in the nails. When liver-blood is deficient, the nails become dark, indented, dry, or cracked.

In Chinese tradition, the liver houses the "ethereal soul," an energy that survives the body at death to flow back into the world of subtle energies. The ethereal soul is said to influence the individual's capacity for life planning and finding purpose in life. When the liver flourishes, the ethereal soul is firmly rooted and can help the individual plan life with wisdom and vision. On a day to day level, the liver houses emotions. When the circulation of the liver's *ki* is obstructed, emotional energy becomes restrained and gives rise to frustration, depression or anger. These may be accompanied by physical symptoms such as abdominal bloating, a heavy feeling in the chest, pain, and a lump in the throat. The energy channels of the liver cross the breast; in women, disturbances of the liver may cause distention of the breasts. The relationship between the liver and the emotional life is reciprocal. Physical impairment of the liver will lead to emotional tension and frustration, and emotional tension and frustration will damage the liver.

Like the other Five Organs, the liver has a relationship to dreams: "When the liver is in excess, one dreams of being angry," records the *Simple Questions*. This book also states, "When the liver is deficient . . . one dreams of lying . . . without being able to get up."

Table 3.2. Herbal Prescriptions for Disturbances of the Liver

Energy Imbalance	Symptoms Including	Formula
Outwardly directed (Yang) energies in excess, containing (Yin) energies in balance	Irregular menstrual periods, hot flashes, restlessness	Augmented Rambling Powder (page 119)
	Cramps, tight neck muscles, mood swings	Bupleurum and Cinnamon Formula (page 222)
	Yeast infections, pelvic inflammation, headache, ringing in the ears, conjunctivitis	Dong Quai and Gentian Powder (page 147)
	Eye pain, headache, memory lapses, nervousness, dizziness	Uncaria Powder (page 211)
Outwardly directed (Yang) energies deficient, containing (Yin) energies in balance	Missed menstrual periods, anemia, fatigue	Combination of Ginseng Formula (page 254) and Dong Quai and Peony Formula (page 150)
Outwardly directed (Yang) energies in balance, containing (Yin) energies deficient	Muscle spasms, cramps, or (in small children) crying fits at night	Licorice, Wheat, and Jujube Formula (page 174)

The literature of Kampo refers to the *heart* as the monarch among organs. It governs the blood and the blood vessels, shows its energies to the world through the tongue, manifests itself in the complexion, and houses the mind.

The Chinese foundations of Kampo taught that the energies of the heart transform the *ki* of food into blood. Healthy heart energies are essential for a proper supply of blood to all the body. When its function is strong, blood is in ample supply and circulation is good, and the person is full of vigor and has a good constitution. The energies of the heart are thought to control the appearance, shape, and color of the tongue, especially the tip of the tongue, as well as the sense of taste. The condition of the heart also affects speech. Abnormalities of the energies of the heart and circulatory system may cause stuttering or aphasia. The heart influences talking and laughing, and a disharmony of the heart can cause incessant talking.

In traditional East Asian medicine, mental activity and consciousness "reside" in the heart. These energies influence the emotions, memory, thinking, and sleep. If the heart is strong and blood is sufficient, there will be normal mental activity. There will be a balanced emotional life, good memory, clear perception, keen thinking and good sleep. If the heart is weak and blood deficient, there may be mental problems. Some heart functions in relation to the mind correspond to the activities modern thinking associates with the brain. Modern herbal support for attention deficit disorder in children, for example, is based on formulas designed to be a tonic to the heart.

Since the heart houses the mind, it is very closely related to sleep. If the heart is weak, the mind is homeless and it will "float" at night, causing excessive dreaming. All dreams are related to the heart, but certain dreams are more indicative of a heart disharmony. The *Simple Questions* record, "When the heart is weak, one dreams of fires." The *Spiritual Axis* (Ling Shu), a series of conversations about linking the energies of heaven, earth, and human beings through acupuncture, says, "When the Heart is in excess, one dreams of laughing . . . when the heart is deficient, one dreams of mountains, fire and smoke."

Table 3.3 Herbal Prescriptions for Disturbances of the Heart

Energy Imbalance	Symptoms Including	Formula
Outwardly directed (Yang) energies in excess, containing (Yin) energies in balance	Red face, quick temper, tendency for bleeding (especially nosebleed), constipation, feeling of heat	Coptis Antidote (page 143)
	Nervousness, insomnia, restlessness, "stomach rumbles," nausea, vomiting, localized fever	Pinellia Draining Formula (page 274)
Outwardly directed (Yang) energies in balance, containing (Yin) energies deficient	Nervousness, irritable bladder, depression, fatigue	Cinnamon, Dragon Bone, and Oyster Shell Formula (page 137)
	Insomnia, physical weakness, mild fever, dry mouth, dry cough, lethargy	Angelica Formula (page 108)
Both outwardly directed (Yang) and containing (Yin) energies deficient, Yang predominates	Tachycardia, shortness of breath, irregular pulse, dry skin, dry mouth, easy fatigue	Honey-Fried Licorice Formula (page 261)

The energies of the *spleen* are those most intimately associated with *ki*. These energies assist the stomach by transporting and transforming the energy essences of food. These essences combine with the air to form a "gathering" of energies and are also the basis of blood. The energy extracted from food by the spleen helps the blood stay in its normal channels. It is refined to power the muscles and the arms and legs, and in the theory of Kampo, houses thought. Energies of the spleen provide a "residence" for the abilities for thinking, studying, concentrating, focusing, and memorizing.

The Yellow Emperor's Canon of Internal Medicine states that the body itself diagnoses abnormalities of the spleen through dreams. Chapter 80 of the *Simple Questions* says, "If the spleen is deficient, one dreams of being hungry; if the dream takes place in late summer, one dreams of building a house." Chapter 43 of the *Spiritual Axis* says, "If the spleen is in excess, one dreams of singing and being very heavy. If the spleen is deficient, one dreams of abysses in mountains and of swamps."

Table 3.4 Herbal Prescriptions for Disturbances of the "Spleen" (Digestive Energies)

Energy Imbalance	Symptoms Including	Formula
Outwardly directed (Yang) energies in deficiency, containing (Yin) energies in balance	Diarrhea without fever or muscle cramps	Cinnamon Formula (page 133)
	Headache, vomiting, occasional diarrhea, "stomach rumbles"	Evodia Formula (page 243)
	Loss of appetite, nausea, vomiting, diarrhea, fatigue, pain in stomach when taking a small amount of food	Four Gentlemen Formula (page 251)
	Heavy feeling in the head, headache, dizziness, intolerance of low temperature, marked fatigue after eating	Uncaria Powder (page 211)
	Occasional diarrhea, pain in the upper abdomen and chest	Ginseng Formula (page 254)
	Pale complexion, memory lapses, insomnia, depression, feeling of heaviness in the stomach	Restore the Spleen Formula (page 276)
	Loss of appetite, bloating, nausea, vomiting, easy fatigue, "stomach rumbles"	Six-Gentlemen Formula (page 280)
Outwardly directed (Yang) and containing (Yin) energies, both deficient, Yang stronger	Sweating at night, fatigue, tension in the abdominal muscles	Astragalus Formula (page 116)
	Pain around the navel, freckling or ane spots appear at same time as digestive symptoms, hot hands and feet	Minor Construct the Middle Formula (page 180)
Outwardly directed (Yang) containing (Yin) energies, equally deficient	Anemia, cold hands and feet, dry or thin skin	Ten-Significant Tonic Decoction (page 202)

The *lungs* govern respiration, control channels and blood vessels, provide the energies that disperse fluids throughout the body and send fluids downward in the body and control the skin and hair. Their energy channels meet the world at the nose. The lungs inhale "pure *ki*" and exhale "dirty *ki*." They are thought to combine food energy with the energy of the air. Because of their role in extracting *ki* from the air, they are the most external of all the organs, and the most subject to pathogenic attack.

The *ki* produced by the lungs is an essential aid to the heart in circulating blood, and is also essential for propelling energy through all the channels. They disperse immune energy throughout the body, especially in to the space between the skin and the muscles. In so doing, they give the skin and hair nourishment and moisture. When the lungs are healthy, the skin is supple and the hair is glossy, and the opening and closing of the pores and perspiration will be normal. Opening into the nose, the lungs energize the sense of smell.

The *Simple Questions* records that "When the lungs are in excess, one dreams of weeping." It also says, "If the lungs are deficient, one will dream of white objects or about blood killings . . . of battles and war." The *Spiritual Axis* records, "When the lungs are in excess, one will have dreams of worry and fear, or crying and flying. If the lungs are deficient, one will dream of flying and seeing strange objects made of gold or iron."

Table 3.5 Herbal Prescriptions for Disturbances of the Lungs

Energy Imbalance	Symptoms Including	Formula
Outwardly directed (Yang) deficient, containing (Yin) energies in balance	Runny nose, cough, sore throat, chills, colds hands and feet	Ephedra, Asiasarum, and Prepared Aconite Formula (page 242)
	Runny nose, foamy sputum, chills, fever, sound of fluctuating liquid in the digestive tract	Minor Bluegreen Dragon Decoction (page 182)
Outwardly directed (Yang) energies in balance, fluids (Yin) deficient	Dry throat, coughing fits, lump in the throat, hiccups	Japanese Lily Formula (page 261)

The Yang and Yin of the *kidneys* are the foundation of Yang and Yin for all the other organs. Kidney-Yang is the motive force of all physiological processes. Kidney-Yin is the basic substance for reproduction, birth, and growth. The kidneys house the "DNA" of the energy body. This energy essence is said to "fill up the brain" and control the bones, teeth, and hair. The energy channels of the kidneys open into the ears and enable hearing.

The kidneys also control the body's reception of *ki*. They lungs direct the *qi* of the air down to the kidneys, which "hold" it. This energy is intimately connected with will power. If the kidneys are strong, the will power is strong, and the mind is focused on goals that it sets for itself and pursues them in a single-minded way. Conversely, if the kidneys are weak, will power will be lacking, and the mind will be easily discouraged.

The Yellow Emperor's Canon of Internal Medicine states that, "When the kidneys are weak, one dreams of swimming after a shipwreck. If the dream takes place in winter, one dreams of plunging in water and being scared." The *Spiritual Axis* states that, "When the Kidneys are in excess, one dreams the spine is detached from the body. When they are weak, one dreams of being immersed in water."

Table 3.6 Herbal Prescriptions for Disturbances of the Kidneys

Energy Imbalance	Symptoms Including	Formula
Outwardly directed (Yang) energies and fluids (Yin), both deficient	Easy fatigue, nocturnal urination, feeling of incomplete urination, lower back pain, reduced abdominal tension in the lower abdomen, sensitivity to cold but hot or sweaty hands and feet, tending toward swelling.	Six-Ingredient Pill with Rehmannia (page 194)

Traditional Chinese Medicine (TCM) as it is practiced today offers a much richer understanding of the body's energy organs. TCM recognizes six paired organs corresponding to the twelve principal meridians, as do other Japanese healing arts, such as acupuncture and shiatsu. East Asian traditional medicine can describe a far more complex and detailed system of energy relationships. These five organs, however, are enough to complete a diagnostic methodology for effective herbal medicines. The simplicity of the Kampo system allows it to be used effectively with any East Asian healing discipline as well as with modern pharmaceutical treatments.

Part II

和漢薬 Introduction:

One Formula, Many Conditions

Kampo is an ancient system of herbal teas that can be used with any traditional healing practice of Eastern Asia. Kampo is also a scientific system of patent medicines, manufactured under safe and secure sanitary conditions, that can be used with or in place of many modern prescription drugs.

Part 2 of this book is a snapshot of the home medicine cabinet of Kampo. These herbal formulas are the way Japanese medicine restores balance to *ki*. They are also the way Japanese medicine, both traditional and modern, stops the symptoms of many diseases. These thirty-six herbal formulas are available as tablets or instant teas from grocers, health-food stores, pharmacies, and practitioners of traditional Asian medicine across the United States and Canada.

These thirty-six herbal formulas treat far more than thirty-six ailments. For the most part, they are what the ancient Japanese referred to as "high class medicine." They are safe, effective, and useful in treating not just one but many health conditions. Their ability to treat multiple diseases derives from the fact that they were originally designed to treat persons, not illnesses. Combinations of herbs treat combinations of symptoms that recur in different health conditions. One formula may treat many different diseases. On the other hand, individuals may have significantly different experiences of the same disease condition as it is defined in medical terms. A single disease condition may be treated with several different formulas. The most useful formula is the one that most closely matches individual symptoms.

To choose the formula that best meets your health needs, begin with the diagnosis provided by your professional health practitioner. As a general rule, any condition that lasts more than a week, and any condition that could result in a medical emergency, requires an exam by a qualified physician, naturopath, or doctor of Oriental medicine. Conditions that have been previously diagnosed by a doctor, and everyday illnesses such as colds and headaches, are suitable for self-diagnosis and self-treatment with Kampo. To turn to the proper formula, you only need to look under your disease condition in the index of this book. In the index you will find entries such as "Colds, with stuffy nose and neck pain," with the page number for the formula that treats that combination of symptoms for that condition.

For each of the formulas listed in Part 2, you will find a complete listing of synonyms and brand names. These are the various Japanese, Chinese, and English names under which the formula is sold in English-speaking countries. Following the list of names are lists of the herbs the formula contains and medical conditions it treats.

Next is a "test question" that will allow you to decide whether the formula meets your unique health needs. Each formula treats a unique combination of symptoms. This combination of symptoms applies to more than one disease. You can use the scoring charts in Chapter 2 to make your own energy diagnosis and determine whether the formula is likely to treat the symptoms you experience. Then, if your physician has given you a diagnosis of one of the medical conditions listed for the formula, and you experience a *majority* of the symptoms the formula treats, the formula will be helpful in controlling your underlying health condition.

Each entry also offers an explanation of each formula as energy medicine. Formulas are described in the same terms as would be used by an acupuncturist or traditional Asian herbalist. Entries also document formulas as scientific medicine, described in terms of pharmacology, physiology, and modern medical practice, with special note made of potential interactions with prescription drugs and other herbal formulas that may be more effective for certain symptoms.

The selection of formula names used in this book was biased to favor plain English. For example, a frequently cited literal translation of a Chinese formula name, "Augmented Restore the Spleen Decoction," was replaced with a simple reference to the main herb in the combination, "Angelica Formula." In general, the term "decoction" (referring to a tea made with boiling water) is not used in this book, since modern Kampo formulas do not have to be made in teapots. When traditional names are used, they are accompanied by explanations of terminology.

The formulas recommended here are highly effective in correcting symptoms of disease. This is due to the fact that Kampo products are manufactured to exacting standards of purity, quality, and safety. Good Manufacturing Practice (GMP) is followed by all Japanese manufacturers of herbal products and is increasingly followed by manufacturers in the People's Republic of China, Taiwan, Hong Kong, and the United States.

Good Manufacturing Practice

The Japanese Ministry of Health and Welfare must certify every Kampo product manufactured in Japan as safe and effective. The same standards apply whether the product is made for export or for local consumption. This fourteen-step process begins when the herbs are harvested in the People's Republic of China and continues for three years after the herbs are bottled, even after the finished product is available to customers from the retail shelf.

The Chinese government no longer allows any herbs to be shipped to Japan without inspection and processing. Prior to the late 1990's, farming collectives sometimes took shortcuts to meet their production quotas. For instance, if a Kampo manufacturer ordered 100 tons of an herb and there was a drought, so that only ninety-five tons of the herb were grown, it was not unusual to find rocks or kindling wood in the bottom of shipping cases. Various kinds of non-herbal materials served to bring the total shipment to the required weight. While these contaminants could be easily removed from the herbs at a relatively small expense to the Kampo makers, the reputation of the Chinese herb growers was damaged. Accordingly, the Chinese government mandated changes in production.

Nowadays, every Japanese Kampo product maker runs a joint venture with a Chinese processing firm. Herbs are inspected under *Japanese* standards before they are graded, sorted, washed, dried, and cut for further processing in Japan. And increasingly, the high standards of Japanese herb product manufacture are being implemented in China as well.

The first step of herb inspection is commonsensical: does the herb "look right?" While experienced buyers have an intuitive feel for herb quality, samples of each shipment are examined under the microscope. If the herb passes visual inspection, then there is a second level of testing. The herb is dried, pulverized, and analyzed by thin-layer chromatography. This color test not only confirms visual identification but also confirms the presence of adequate concentrations of active chemical ingredients in the herb. Every lot of herbs submitted for manufacture undergoes this test.

Once the herb and its chemical constituents are authenticated, technicians test the product for heavy metal contamination. Heavy metals do not have to be completely absent from the herb. The *Japanese Pharmacopoeia* permits lead in concentrations of up to 30 parts per million and arsenic in concentrations of up to 2 parts per million. Since US standards are stricter for lead (10 parts per million), Japanese companies exporting to the US have adopted a more stringent test for lead contamination. The Japanese limits for heavy metals other than lead are stricter than those used in the United States. Other quality control steps ensure that herbs are properly dried and contain only traces of ash caused by scorching the herbs during the drying process.

The formulas of Kampo were originally taken as teas. Their modern counterparts are essentially tablets of "instant tea." At the factory, chopped herbs are mixed with twenty times their weight in purified water. The mixture is gradually warmed over a period of forty minutes to a temperature just below boiling and then allowed to steep for one hour. Then the tea is strained through a mesh and the liquid portion sprayed in a low-pressure chamber at a temperature of 100° F (approximately 40° C) or less until the extract powder falls out. The resulting powder is then dried. Its volume is about the same as the volume of the raw herbs.

The same quality control steps performed on the raw herbs are repeated on the herb extract. The extract is tested for heavy metals and arsenic. The active chemical compounds found in the herbs must also be found in the herb extract.

The next step in the manufacturing process is to mix the herb extract with a carrier to be molded into tablets. The tablets are extruded individually to be put in bottles or placed in a plastic bubble sheet for individual dosing. Even at this point, quality control continues. The Japanese government requires manufactures to show that the content of Kampo products does not change even under severe conditions, roughly equivalent to storing the tablets in the glove compartment of a car during the summer in a humid climate for six months. Products are required to be stable at room temperature for three years.

In a typical stability test, the amount of an active chemical in a daily dose of Kampo might degrade by 0.5 percent at room temperature or 2-3 percent under severe conditions when stored for six months. When the formula is preserved as a tincture, the loss of active ingredients is about half as great.

GMP answers many of the important concerns of physicians and pharmacists about the use of herbal medicine. Herbs are known to exert their effects due to a number of ingredients working in concert. GMP makes sure that every herb product includes all of the herb's most important constituents. Critics of herbal medicine also point out that even standardized products could vary from manufacturer to manufacturer. Every manufacturer in Japan, however, standardizes Kampo products in exactly the same way. These procedures make Japanese herbal medicines as predictable as prescription drugs.

Aconite

Japanese Name: Kakobushi-matsu (pure aconite), *Bushi-to* (aconite with other herbs)
Chinese Name: Zhi Chuan Wu (medication containing pure aconite), Fu Zi Li Zhong Tang (aconite with other herbs)
Scientific Name: Formula aconiti

Common Brand Names

Aconite Combination (Brion)
Aconite, Ginger, and Ginseng Combination (Lotus Classics, Sun Ten)

Aconite, Ginger, and Licorice Combination (Lotus Classics)
Aconite, Ginseng, and Ginger (Qualiherb)
Bushi-to (Honso,* Tsumura*)
Fu Zi Li Zhong Tang (Lotus Classics, Qualiherb, Sun Ten)
Kakobushi-matsu (Honso,* Tsumura*)
(* Made in Japan.)

Herbs Used to Make a Single Dose

Aconite tuber in various amounts, which may be combined with white atractylodis, ginseng, peony root, and/or poria mushroom.

Health Conditions Treated

Symptomatic relief of autoimmune diseases including Grave's disease, insulin-dependent diabetes, lupus, multiple sclerosis, rheumatoid arthritis, and Sjögren's syndrome.

Who Should Use This Formula?

Persons with chronic health conditions causing physical weakness, sensation of coldness, shortness of breath, and fatigue. Persons who have fever should never use this formula.

Consider this formula if you have any of the health conditions listed above and experience

Pain and cold throughout the body, scanty urination, swelling (ascites, edema), shortness of breath, and/or swollen joints. Japanese physicians recommend this formula to weak, exhausted patients with coldness and pain throughout the entire body, under the care of both a physician and a trained practitioner of East Asian medicine. This herb should never be self-prescribed, and is not for use by children or during pregnancy.

Energy Diagnosis

This formula is appropriate for an energy diagnosis of:

- Either Second or Sixth Stage of Disease
- *Ki* deficiency
- Yin state with cold.

Explanation

Japanese physicians cautiously prescribe aconite when a patient with a chronic autoimmune disease has taken a sudden turn for the worse. Autoimmune diseases are the result of the immune system's mistaken coding of an antibody or a T cell to attack the body itself rather than an infectious microorganism. As long as the immune system is not activated, the autoimmune condition is not troubling. However, most health conditions in this category can change rapidly when some outside trigger causes the immune system to produce large quantities of antibodies or T cells. Disease-fighting antibodies and T cells and self-destructive antibodies and T cells are both produced in huge quantities in response to infection. Unchecked, errant immune cells can attack specific organs or even the entire body.

The immune system goes on to produce a cascade of inflammatory reactions that destroy tissues and interfere with the metabolism. Weakness, exhaustion, and an overwhelming feeling of cold ensue. A peculiarity of autoimmune diseases is that this especially destructive phase of the condition can act simultaneously with the everyday problems they cause. The day to day joint pain of rheumatoid arthritis, for instance, does not go away when the disease attacks the kidneys.

Even worse, in many autoimmune diseases, pain itself causes tissue destruction. In the healthy body, nerves known as nociceptors release Substance P (for pain), which signals white blood cells to "clear out" infected or injured tissues. Unfortunately the nociceptors can also be activated by the pain of autoimmune disease to "clear out" healthy tissues. This is a special problem of rheumatoid arthritis.

The ancient masters of energy medicine were familiar with autoimmune diseases. They described a condition in which the disease "jumped" from the Second Stage of Disease, in which the body has begun to fight an infection with immune cells rather than just sweating and fever, directly to the Sixth Stage of Disease, in which the body's vital energies are depleted. They also described situations in which the two stages of disease seem to operate simultaneously. That is, while the body as a whole might be depleted of energy, there still might be enough Yang energy in the "outer layers" of the body to cause joint pain, fever, and rashes.

Kampo physicians gave aconite, the most Yang of all herbs, when the need to re-energize the body greatly outweighed the risk of causing joint pain, fever, and skin outbreaks. Because of the potential toxic effects of the herb, aconite was and is only given for the most severe symptoms. Herbal authorities note that any beneficial effects of aconite should be noticed within one to three hours of administration.

Documentation

The Yang of Aconite derives from a potent analgesic agent, mesaconitine. This chemical raises the threshold of pain and helps the body regulate itself in conditions of either stress or relaxation. Mesaconitine manipulations the brain's production of norepinephrine, one of the chemicals that "excites" the nerve cells that release Substance P. It increases the central nervous system's production of norepinephrine during stress, and it decreases the central nervous system's production of norepinephrine[1] to allow relaxation.

Pure mesaconitine is a more potent pain reliever than morphine. Another compound found in aconite, lappaconitine, has eight times the analgesic effect of cocaine on mucous membranes.[2] The whole processed aconite tuber these chemicals come from is about as effective in relieving pain as indomethacin, the pain-relieving ingredient in Advil and Motrin.[3] The advantage of using aconite over using Advil or Motrin lies in its ability to stimulate circulation, raise body temperature, and stop vomiting and diarrhea.

Interactions with Other Nutritional Supplements

Aconite indirectly increases the effectiveness of glucosamine by preventing tissue breakdown in rheumatoid arthritis. However, aconite is not suitable for long-term use.

Comparisons to Other Formulas

Aconite is sometimes used to "jump start" the metabolism. Kampo practitioners use aconite to increase the effectiveness of Peony and Licorice Decoction, Gypsum and Atractylodis Formula, or Ginseng Formula.

Warning: Although aconite tinctures are available without prescription from herbalists and in some retail stores, never use this herb without expert advice. Aconite in therapeutic dosages may cause temporary numbness of the tongue and lips. Paralysis of lips and tongue, racing heart, feeling of uprising heat, or redness in the face are signs of overdose and require immediate medical care. The medical antidotes for aconite poisoning are atropine, procaine, and glucocorticoids, which can only be administered by a physician.

Angelica Formula

This formula is also known as Augmented Restore the Spleen Decoction. The traditional name of this formula refers to its ability to restore the ability of the "spleen," or the energies of digestion, to control the flow of blood.

Japanese Name: Kami-kihi-to
Chinese Name: Jia Wei Gui Pi Tang
Scientific Name: Formula lienalis angelicae compositae

Common Brand Names

Ginseng & Longan Comb. Mod. (Qualiherb)
Ginseng, Longan, & Bupleurum Combination (Sun Ten)
Jia Wei Gui Pi Tang (Qualiherb, Sun Ten)
Kami-kihi-to (Honso,* Tsumura*)
(*Made in Japan)

Herbs Used to Make a Single Dose

Ginseng 3.0 g
White Atractylodis Root 3.0 g
Poria 3.0 g
Astragalus Root 3.0 g
Angelica Root 2.0 g
Polygala Root 2.0 g
Bupleurum Root 3.0 g
Cornelian Cherry Fruit 2.0 g
Licorice Root 1.0 g
Saussurea Root 1.0 g
Jujube Fruit 2.0 g
Ginger (dried) 1.0 g
Cornelian Cherry Fruit 3.0 g
Longan Fruit 3.0 g

Health Conditions Treated

Emotional conditions:: adult ADD/ADHD, anemia, anxiety, and insomnia.

Skin conditions: bruising, allergic purpura, thrombocytopenic purpura, and vitiligo.

Who Should Use This Formula?

Physically weak individuals who experience anemia and/or emotional fatigue.

Consider This Formula If You Have Any of the Health Conditions Listed Above and Experience

Fatigue, emotional or physical weakness, tendency for fear, or unexplained neurological symptoms (twitches, memory lapses, fainting spells).

Energy Diagnosis

This formula is appropriate for an energy diagnosis of:

- Second Stage of Disease
- *Ki* neither deficient nor excessive

Explanation

"The way to a man's heart is through his stomach" used to be a frequently quoted saying in the English language. The Japanese language has even more expressions linking the emotions with the *hara*, or stomach. *Hara ga tatsu* roughly translates as "That gets me in the gut," meaning "I am angry." The term *hara-hara*, which might be literally (and incorrectly) translated as "stomach-stomach," means fear. And the expression *hara ga mieseku*, "your stomach is showing," means one's intentions are obvious.

The intimate interrelationship between the digestive system and the brain has also been recognized in modern medicine. Serotonin is considered to be the key chemical for maintaining mood. The commonly prescribed antidepressants Prozac, Paxil, and Zoloft act by regulating serotonin. Over ninety-five percent of the body's supply of this chemical, however, is found in the digestive system.

The digestive tract uses serotonin to signal the brain when something is wrong. Food poisoning, for example, causes the stomach's enterochromaffin cells to pour out massive quantities of serotonin, which tells the brain to start a vomiting reflex. Antidepressant treatment that increases the amount of serotonin in the brain also increases the amount of serotonin in the intestines and can also trigger the vomiting reflex. Conversely, too little serotonin in the digestive tract can cause constipation and a "locked" digestive tract.

While Prozac, Paxil, and Zoloft were of course unknown in ancient Asia, Kampo medicine also treated imbalances between the processes of thought and digestion. Continuous intellectual activity was thought to cause the person to become "ungrounded," and thereby injure the Earth organ, the spleen (which corresponds to the digestive tract rather than to the organ identified in modern medicine as the spleen). The spleen is the organ that transforms food into blood. When it is injured, blood becomes deficient and the spleen cannot feed the heart.

The spleen was thought to store intelligence, while the heart was thought to be the home of the spirit. Disturbances of intelligence and spirit lead to anxiety, phobia, insomnia, and dream-disturbed sleep. Blood deficiency may also lead to feverishness associated with heat from deficiency.

The herbs in this formula were chosen to restore the spleen's ability to produce blood. They restore its ability to produce the *ki* of blood, which is important to thought processes and emotional balance. They also renew its ability to produce blood as a physical substance. This is important to correcting anemia, a deficiency of red blood cells, and various forms of purpura, the purple blotching of the skin caused by deficiencies of clotting factors.

Documentation

This formula has been used to treat symptoms in "pensive" individuals since the Song Dynasty of China (960-1279). Laboratory testing has found that it counteracts chemicals that inhibit serotonin, which stimulates mood in the brain and movement in the digestive tract. It also counteracts inflammatory responses to chronic pain.[1]

A clinical study of Angelica Formula for treating purpura conducted in Japan suggests that it will either work quite well, or not work at all. The formula is effective when certain classes of antibodies are found in the blood, and not effective when other classes of antibodies are found in the blood.[2] However, since there are no reported side effects from the use of the formula in clinical treatment, a thirty-day test of the formula in treating purpura is appropriate for anyone with the disease.

Interactions with Other Nutritional Supplements

Angelica Formula will counteract yohimbine.

Comparisons to Other Formulas

Cinnamon and Formula may be more effective when there is no fever and predominant symptoms are fear and restlessness.

Coptis Antidote Formula is preferable when there is general nervousness or excitement, a feeling of heat in the whole body, and widespread muscle tension. In Japan, physicians sometimes use Coptis Antidote Formula to treat the manic stage of bipolar disorder.

Ten-Significant Tonic Decoction may be more effective if there is coldness in hands and feet, tendency for fever, and/or irritability.

Artemisia Yinchenhao and Five-Ingredient Powder with Poria

The term *yinchenhao* refers to the species of artemisia used in this formula, *Artemisia capillaris.*

Japanese Name: Inchin-gorei-san
Chinese Name: Wei Ling Tang
Scientific Name: Pulvis qinque-medicamentorum artemisiae capillaris

Common Brand Names

Inchin-gorei-san (Honso,* Tsumura*)
Magnolia & Hoelen Combination (Lotus Classics, Qualiherb)
(*Made in Japan)

Herbs Used to Make a Single Dose

Alisma Rhizome 6.0 g
White Atractylodis Rhizome 4.5 g
Polyporus 4.5 g
Poria 4.5 g
Cinnamon Bark 2.5 g
Artemisia Spikes 4.0 g

Health Conditions Treated

Diarrhea, dizziness, headache, heartburn, hives, mouth sores.

Symptomatic relief of choledyskinesia, cirrhosis of the liver, gallstones, acute and chronic hepatitis, and nephritis.

Who Should Use This Formula?

Japanese physicians typically recommend this formula to physically active individuals whose symptoms include dehydration, failure to drink adequate fluids, and dry mouth.

Consider This Formula If You Have Any of the Health Conditions Listed Above and Experience

Dry mouth, failure to take fluids, jaundice, loss of appetite, abdominal swelling, stomach rumbles, headache, dizziness. This formula may be appropriate if the abdomen is swollen but is not tight.

Energy Diagnosis

This formula is appropriate for an energy diagnosis of:

- Second Stage of Disease
- Depressed or static *ki*

Explanation

Kampo medicine defines the *sho* (symptom pattern) for this formula as a manifestation of the Second Stage of Disease, in which the invading illness has penetrated the body's outermost defenses. In the First Stage of Disease, the body attempted to "sweat out" the illness with perspiration, tightening the muscles and blood vessels to keep the disease from progressing inward. This activity requires an ample supply of blood flowing to the outer layers of the body. If enough blood does not reach the outer layers, the immune response is weaker.

In this symptom pattern, the disease influence is too strong for the first level of defenses. It progresses to the Greater Yang organ, the bladder. There it attacks and disrupts the functions of the bladder, resulting in difficult urination. Disrupting bladder function also leads to water retention, which interferes with upward transformation and downward elimination of fluids. Fluids that cannot be transported at all cause swelling in the abdomen. Fluids that resist transportation cause rumbling in the stomach. Fluids that are transported up rather than down cause vomiting and heartburn. The body's Yang energies are bottled up in the bladder. They do not reach the head, causing dizziness and headache.

This scenario first described in the second century by the father of Kampo, Zhang Zhong-jing. Surprisingly, it has a correlate in modern medicine. The most current explanation of the phenomenon of ascites, or swollen abdomen, is that hardened tissues in the liver cause the portal vein serving it to become filled with blood and the blood pressure in that vein to become high. The bottling up of blood in the portal vein takes blood away from other vessels, which signal the kidneys that blood pressure overall is too low. To make up for the "missing" blood volume, the kidneys retain fluid even though the body's supply blood is not low. The resulting fluid leaks out of the blood vessels and causes abdominal swelling.

The symptom pattern for this formula specifies that the body's overall condition of *ki* is neither deficient nor excessive. Therefore, Artemisia and Poria Five-Ingredient Powder is designed to redirect energies rather than to stimulate them. The two mushrooms in this formula, polyporus and poria, are included in many formulas to move water by promoting urination. The venerable Zhang Zhong-jing included cinnamon to "light a fire under the cauldron" and help the

Yang energies of the body move upward as needed, preventing headache and dizziness. Artemisia is included for its specific immune-stimulant effects and to relieve liver conditions.

Documentation

Most of the research efforts concerning this formula have focused on just one herb, artemisia. A pilot study in China found that about two-thirds of hepatitis B patients given artemisia experience reduced levels of liver damage after one year on the formula.[1] Laboratory studies have also found artemisia stops the reproduction of human liver cancer cells in the test tube. The most recent reports from Taiwan suggest that artemisia has "significant" antiviral effects on HIV. All of these studies are preliminary, however, and conclusive findings are lacking.

The two medicinal mushrooms in the formula, poria and polyporus, are well documented to stimulate urination. Japanese studies of all the herbs in Artemisia and Poria Five-Ingredient Powder *except* artemisia offer a second explanation of how the formula may relieve water retention. In a laboratory investigation, an extract of the herbs was added to smooth muscle tissue like that lining the arteries. The muscle fibers contracted.[2] In the human body, "loose" linings of arteries cause fluid retention, so this mechanism may explain the formula's ability to relieve abdominal swelling.

Interactions with Commonly Prescribed Drugs

Although Artemisia and Poria Five-Ingredient Powder has not been scientifically examined for potential drug interactions, the arterial contraction studies suggest that it would counteract the prescription drug Viagra (sildenafil).

Comparisons to Other Formulas

Bupleurum and Poria Formula is a preferred alternative when there is tenderness on the right side of the abdomen.

Calm the Stomach and Poria Formula is a preferred alternative when there is diarrhea and gas.

Astragalus Formula

This formula is also known as Astragalus Decoction to Construct the Middle. This formula's traditional name refers to its ability to build up *ki* in the middle of the body, stopping cramps in the stomach and abdomen.

Japanese Name: Ogi-kenchu-to
Chinese Name: Huang Qi Jian Zhong Tang
Scientific Name: Formula astragali

Common Brand Names
Astragalus Formula (Golden Flower)
Huang Qi Jian Zhong Tang (Lotus Classics, Qualiherb, Sun Ten)
Ogi-kenchu-to (Honso,* Tsumura*)
(*Made in Japan)

Herbs Used to Make a Single Dose
Peony 6.0 g
Jujube Fruit 4.0 g
Astragalus Root 4.0 g
Licorice Root 4.0 g
Cinnamon Bark 2.0 g
Ginger (fresh) 1.0 g

Traditionally, each dose of this formula was taken with an ounce (30 g) of sugar. Chinese-made patent medicines based on this formula sometimes include sugar, but Japanese-made products do not.

Health Conditions Treated
Acute symptoms of allergies, gastritis, gastric ulcers, inflamma-

tory bowel disease, and peptic ulcers. Chronic symptoms of boils, dermatitis, eczema, and wounds that fail to heal.

Who Should Use This Formula?

Physically inactive individuals who tire easily.

Consider This Formula If You Have Any of the Health Conditions Listed Above and Experience

Exhaustion, night sweats, loss of appetite, shortness of breath, periodic attacks of eczema, loss of appetite, and/or tightness of abdominal muscles.

Energy Diagnosis

This formula is appropriate for an energy diagnosis of:

- Fourth Stage of Disease
- Excessive Yin
- *Ki* deficiency

Explanation

Astragalus Formula is a variation on a combination of herbs the venerable third-century doctor Zhang Zhong-jing gave to treat "vexation." In this condition, various emotional and environmental frustrations gradually deplete the energies of the body. They eventually overcome the Yang, the body's outwardly directed energies.

By the time boils, dermatitis, eczema, or open wounds become chronic, or allergies, gastritis, gastric or peptic ulcers, or inflammatory bowel disease become recurrent, these "vexations" have lodged in the middle energy layers of the body. The digestive function or the "spleen" is particularly affected. The purpose of the formula is restore Yang energies and revitalize the immune system and digestive function. Properly energized, the "spleen" can then send energy to the muscles, flesh, and skin to cure chronic inflammations or lesions, such as those of dermatitis, eczema, or open wounds.

This formula is especially gentle. It is frequently recommended for children, especially in treating chronic allergies that cause skin inflammation and allergies associated with chronic ear infections.

Documentation

The writings of Zhang Zhong-jing are very clear that Astragalus Formula treats vexations in the heart. Clinical research in China has confirmed that astragalus improves circulation after a heart attack by increasing the action of the left ventricle, the heart's main pumping chamber.[1] Astragalus increases the effectiveness of lidocaine, commonly prescribed to prevent a weak, erratic heartbeat called ventricular fibrillation.[2] The herb also protects heart tissues from damage after circulation is restored following a heart attack or bypass surgery.[3]

The traditional uses of this formula have also been confirmed by research that finds that its herbs release chemicals that signal the brain to release three proteins that control digestion and motion in the intestines. These proteins are gastrin, motilin, and somatostatin.[4] Gastrin controls the steady secretion of gastric juices needed to digest proteins. The irritant chemical histamine can intermingle with gastrin to cause the stomach to churn out large quantities of acidic gastric juices, but the licorice in the formula counteracts the release of histamine. In this way Astragalus Formula halts the release of quantities of stomach acid large enough to initiate or aggravate ulcers. Somatostatin allows the release of bicarbonate (the active ingredient in bicarbonate of soda) from the pancreas and prevents spasms of the gallbladder. Once this bicarbonate has been released, motilin makes the muscles of the upper gastrointestinal tract contract to move food downward to the intestine out of the stomach quickly, with a minimal amount of acid.

In addition to stopping excessive production of acid in the stomach, the ginger and ginseng formula activate other muscles to ensure smooth transit of digested food through the intestine.[5] The ginger in the formula helps prevent severe constipation in people coming off morphine or Vicodin,[6] and the astragalus helps maintain a healthy bacterial balance in the intestine.[7]

Medical science has not confirmed that traditional use of this formula in treating vitiligo, but it is known that the formula induces the immune system to produce the hormone interleukin-2 IL-2.[8] A synthetic form of IL-2 is sometimes used in the medical treatment of vitiligo.

Comparisons to Other Formulas

When there are "cold" symptoms, such as severe diarrhea or an ongoing perception of cold, Minor Construct the Middle Formula may be more effective.

Augmented Rambling Powder

This formula takes its name from an ancient Daoist teaching known as wu wei, the path of no action. Wu and Wei were also names of two princes of the land reached on a happy excursion to nowhere in a famous short story in Chinese literature. Rather than "no action," this formula offers jia wei, or "energetic action," allowing the user to ramble down life's path unencumbered. The Japanese name of the formula is a play on words that could be interpreted as "fortified powder for life's easy walk," referring to the fact it adds herbs to a basic formula. Alternatively, the Japanese name for this formula at one time meant "fortifying powder for life's easy walk," referring to its ability to give women added energy to deal with health problems.

Japanese Name: Kami-shoyo-san
Chinese Name: Jia Wei Shao Yao San
Scientific Name: Pulvis titubationis compositae

Common Brand Names

Bupleurum & Peony Formula (Lotus Classics, Qualiherb, Sun Ten)

Free and Easy Wanderer Plus (Golden Flower)
Jia Wei Xiao Yao San (Lotus Classics, Qualiherb, Sun Ten)
Kami-shoyo-san (Tsumura*)
Kampo4WomenMindEase (Honso*)
(*Made in Japan)

Herbs Used to Make a Single Dose

Bupleurum Root 3.0 g
Peony Root 3.0 g
Angelica Root 3.0 g
Poria 3.0 g
Cornelian Cherry Fruit 2.0 g
Moutan Root 2.0 g
Licorice Root 1.5 g
Ginger (fresh) 1.0 g
Mint Leaf and Stems 1.0 g
White Atractylodis Rhizome 3.0 g

Health Conditions Treated

In women: Symptomatic relief of fatigue, painful tension of the shoulder and neck muscles, anxiety, insomnia, constipation, and missed or scanty periods. Relieves hot flashes, insomnia, and irritability in women taking drugs to lower estrogen levels to treat endometriosis and or to lower testosterone levels to treat hirsutism (excessive body hair).

Who Should Use This Formula?

Women who experience fatigue, painful tension of the shoulder and neck muscles, anxiety, insomnia, constipation, and/or missed or scanty periods.

Consider This Formula If You Have Any of the Health Conditions Listed Above and Experience

Marked fatigue with restless, fearfulness, insomnia, and/or irritability; perception of cold in the lower part of the body, painful tension in shoulder and neck muscles, abdominal cramps, redness of the skin, unexplained sweating, periodic dizziness, headaches, and/or skin outbreaks beginning with menstrual period.

Energy Diagnosis

This formula is appropriate for an energy diagnosis of:

- Second Stage of Disease
- *Ki* deficiency
- *Oketsu* syndrome

Explanation

Japanese physicians explain the conditions this formula treats as a drain of Yang energies resulting in the *oketsu* syndrome. Constantly responding to emotional stress, or constantly responding to food-borne infections, women's energies are depleted. When stress comes from these two sources, the liver is especially vulnerable. It loses its ability to send blood where it needs to go in the body. This is the condition known as *oketsu*. This syndrome is marked by hot flashes, muscle pain, lumbago, darkened pigment in the skin and circles under the eyes, spasms of peripheral blood vessels, and painful hemorrhoids. It also causes missed periods, coldness, tension, and skin outbreaks. *The Imperial Grace Formulary of the Tai Ping Era* (an ancient textbook of Kampo) goes on to say that constant emotional stress in women eventually "steams the bones," leading to arthritis and immobility.

Documentation

A more modern explanation of how this formula works is that it regulates the action of estrogen so that too much or too little of the hormone does not necessarily result in unpleasant symptoms. A study of thirteen women experiencing drug-induced menopause at the Osaka City University Medical School in Japan found that all thirteen obtained relief of hot flashes, insomnia, and mood swings when given this formula or a very similar combination of herbs. Augmented

Rambling Powder does not raise estrogen levels.[1] Instead, it seems to make the estrogen that is available to the body work more effectively.

Augmented Rambling Powder also has some applications in treating diseases of men. Another Japanese study found that the formula stopped tremors in five out of eight patients taking antipsychotic drugs.[2]

Comparisons to Other Formulas

Bupleurum, Dragon Bone, and Oyster Shell Formula may be more effective when the primary symptoms of concern are anxiety, fearfulness, insomnia, and/or irritability.

Bupleurum and Magnolia Formula

Japanese Name: Saiboku-to
Chinese Name: Chai Hu Hou Po Tang
Scientific Name: Formula bupleuri et magnoliae

Common Brand Names

Saiboku-to (Honso,* Tsumura*)
(*Made in Japan)

The raw herbs in this formula are available for use as teas from most Chinese pharmacies and doctors of Oriental medicine. Be careful that any product you are offered contains magnolia bark (*hou po*), which is essential to the action of the formula.

Herbs Used to Make a Single Dose

Bupleurum Root 7.0 g
Pinellia Tuber 5.0 g
Poria 5.0 g

Scutellaria Root 3.0 g
Magnolia Bark 3.0 g
Jujube Fruit 3.0 g
Ginseng 3.0 g
Licorice Root 2.0 g
Perilla Leaf and Stem 2.0 g
Ginger (fresh) 1.0 g

Health Conditions Treated

Asthma in children, bronchitis, colds, chronic gastritis, and lymphedema. Japanese physicians frequently recommend this formula for strengthening weak immune systems in children and teenagers.

Who Should Use This Formula?

Persons whose lifestyle is not impeded by symptoms of disease.

Consider This Formula If You Have Any of the Health Conditions Listed Above and Experience

Wheezing, coughing, tendency toward depression, poor appetite, fatigue, lump in the throat, palpitations, and/or dizziness.

Energy Diagnosis

This formula is appropriate for an energy diagnosis of:

- Second Stage of Disease
- *Ki* stasis. While the energy of the liver and lungs is static, the overall *ki* of the body is neither deficient nor excessive.

Explanation

Bupleurum and Magnolia Formula was designed for a unique combination of symptoms in the Second Stage of Disease. In this symptom pattern, the invading pathogenic energy has managed to "bottle up" *ki* in the lungs and liver. Energy stasis in the lungs expresses itself as labored breathing, wheezing, or congestion. Energy cannot rise to the throat, so there is either hoarseness or a feeling of a lump in the throat.

Energy stasis in the liver expresses itself as emotional constraint and feeling uptight and anxious all the time. The skeletal muscles over the liver on the right side are tense. The energy of positive emotions stored in the liver cannot reach the lungs to ease breathing.

Documentation

While the energy explanation of this formula may seem quaint, the herbs in the formula have been extensively researched. At the end of 2001, no fewer than forty-eight published studies offered scientific documentation of the efficacy of the formula in laboratory and clinical settings. This makes Bupleurum and Magnolia one of the best-studied herbal preparations in the world, although the clinical trials were reported in Japanese-language medical journals that are not indexed on MedLine.

Research interest in this formula began in 1982, when Japanese researchers working with animals found that it could stop both type I allergic reactions (immediate allergic reactions, such as those in asthma) and type IV allergic reactions (delayed allergic reactions, such as those in contact dermatitis). The researchers also found that the formula made it possible to stop allergic reactions with smaller dosages of hydrocortisone.[1]

This finding led to clinical trials in both Japan and the Slovak Republic. In 1985, Japanese physicians published findings from a clinical study of the use of Bupleurum and Magnolia Formula in treating twenty-nine asthma patients. Fifteen patients went into complete remission from asthma after taking the formula for three months. Thirteen patients were able to control their attacks while taking less than half as much steroid medication.[2] Researchers found that the formula kept steroid asthma medications from breaking down, so that smaller doses were equally effective.[3] These findings were repeated by a clinic in Bratislava in what was then Czechoslovakia.

A follow-up study published in the *Annals of the New York Academy of Sciences* in 1993 found that another way the formula helped control asthma was to keep the body from building resistance to asthma medications. When used for six to twelve months, Bupleurum and Magnolia Formula stopped the "downregulation" of steroid drugs. It also stopped allergic reactions to dust mites.[4] Another study published the same year found that whether or not the formula worked depended on the ability of the patient's body to absorb the chemicals released by magnolia bark. That is, magnolia bark was found to be an essential component of the formula.[5]

The most recent research of this formula confirms that it relieves anxiety without causing drowsiness or sedation. While Bupleurum and Magnolia Formula has some of the same beneficial effects as tranquilizers in the same class as Valium and Librium, it does not act on the same sites in the brain and it does not interfere with the body's metabolism of these drugs.[6] Studies at the Tsumura Laboratories and Gumnam University School of Medicine in Japan, and at the University of Texas at San Antonio, confirmed that magnolia bark is the source of the chemicals in the formula that relieve anxiety.[7]

Interactions with Prescription Drugs

Of the millions of people who have taken this formula, approximately ten have developed pneumonia while taking both Bupleurum and Magnolia Formula and interferon treatment without adequate medical supervision. The formula seems to increase the effectiveness of interferon, so that white blood cells accumulate in the lungs and cause severe inflammation. Do not use Bupleurum and Magnolia Formula if you receive interferon therapy, and see a physician immediately if you develop breathing difficulties while taking these herbs.

Never take this formula if your physician has recently increased the dosage of your asthma medications. On the other hand, this formula is particularly helpful for asthmatics whose physicians reduce the dosage of their medications.

Comparisons to Other Formulas

This formula is sometimes given with both Minor Bupleurum Decoction and Pinellia and Magnolia Bark Formula. Minor Bluegreen

Dragon Decoction may be more effective if there is foamy phlegm and nasal irritation is a prominent symptom.

Bupleurum and Poria Formula

Japanese Name: Sairei-to
Chinese Name: Niuche Shen Qi Tang
Scientific Name: Formula bupleuri et hoelen

Common Brand Names
Sairei-to (Tsumura*)

Bupleurum and Poria Formula is a combination of two formulas, Five-Ingredient Powder with Poria and Minor Bupleurum Decoction. Although Bupleurum and Poria Formula is not widely available as a single mixture, it is possible to get the same effect by taking recommended doses of both formulas.

Brand names for Five-Ingredient Powder:
Drain Dampness (Health Concerns)
Sairei-to (Tsumura*)
Hoelen 5 (Chinese Classics)
Hoelen 5-Herb Combination (Qualiherb)
Kampo4Digestive Intestine Harmony (Honso*)
Poria 5 (Golden Flower Chinese Herbs)
Water's Way (Kan Traditionals)
Wu Ling San (Chinese Classics, Golden Flower Chinese Herbs, Kan Traditionals, Lotus Classics, Qualiherb, Sun Ten)

Brand names for Minor Bupleurum Decoction:
Liver Kampo (Honso*)

Minor Bupleurum Combination (Lotus Classics, Qualiherb, Sun Ten)

Minor Bupleurum Formula (Chinese Classics, Golden Flower Chinese Herbs)

Minor Bupleurum Formulation (Kan Traditionals)

Sho-saiko-to (Tsumura*)

Xiao Chai Hu Tang (Lotus Classics, Qualiherb, Sun Ten)

(*Made in Japan)

Components

Bupleurum Root 7.0 g
Alisma Rhizome 5.0 g
Pinellia Tuber 5.0 g
Scutellaria Root 3.0 g
White Atractylodis Rhizome 3.0 g
Jujube Fruit 3.0 g
Polyporus 3.0 g
Ginseng 3.0 g
Poria 3.0 g
Licorice Root 2.0 g
Cinnamon Bark 2.0 g
Ginger (fresh) 1.0 g

Health Conditions Treated

Gastritis, chronic hepatitis, cirrhosis of the liver, nephritis, Ménière's disease, middle ear infections, rheumatoid arthritis, sunstroke.

Who Should Use This Formula?

People whose lifestyle has not been inhibited by their chronic disease.

Consider This Formula If You Have Any of the Health Conditions Listed Above and Experience

Swelling, thirst, scanty urination, loss of appetite, nausea, vomiting, diarrhea, abdominal pain, headache, dizziness, mild fever, tendency to bite one's tongue, and/or "stomach rumbles."

Energy Diagnosis

This formula is appropriate for an energy diagnosis of:

- Second Stage of Disease
- *Ki* neither deficient nor excessive

Explanation

This formula is based on a Kampo combination devised by the master Zhang Zhong-jing, who taught a theory of "half-exterior, half-interior" diseases. In this Second Stage of Disease, the disease-causing energy has weakened but not entirely overcome the basic defenses of the body. Sometimes "right *ki*" prevails, and there is a feeling of heat radiating out of the body to "sweat out" the disease. Sometimes "evil *ki*" prevails, and there is a sensation of chilling cold. As the immune system teeters on the brink of deficiency, symptoms of heat and cold alternate unpredictably and rapidly, several times a day.

Dr. Zhang described a variety of symptoms that modern medicine associates with rheumatoid arthritis, lupus (especially lupus-causing kidney damage), Ménière's disease, rheumatoid arthritis, and sunstroke. If the pathogenic evil persists, Zhang wrote, "the person suffers from fullness in the chest and rib-side, taciturnity (that is, social withdrawal), lack of desire for food and drink, heart vexation and frequent retching, or possibly vexation in the chest and no retching, or thirst and pain in the abdomen, or palpitations below the heart with inhibited urination, or perhaps absence of thirst with generalized heat, or cough." In these cases, Zhang recommended treatment with formulas containing the herb bupleurum.

Documentation

The scientific study of Bupleurum and Poria Formula began in the 1980s when it was investigated for treating chronic ear infections. Physicians at the Tohoku University School of Medicine in Sendai, Japan, gave Bupleurum and Poria Formula to thirty-five children with chronic otitis media for four weeks. While only four cases showed complete remission of symptoms, about seventy percent showed a partial improvement without serious side effects.[1] Physicians at Japan's Keio University then tested the formula as a treatment for adult hearing loss. In cases that respond to steroid treatments, Bupleurum and Poria enabled physicians to prevent further hearing loss, especially for lower frequencies, with an average eighty percent reduction in medication. The herbal formula did not, however, completely replace steroid drugs.[2]

A research effort sponsored by Tsumura & Company in the United States then tested the efficacy of the formula in treating rheumatoid arthritis (RA). Researchers at the University of Utah and UCLA found that twenty percent of RA patients responded to the formula. These patients experienced reduced joint tenderness, pain, and swelling, as well as increased mobility.[3] While this response percentage seems low, it is comparable to the response rate to conventional prescription drugs for RA.

More recent research has focused on Bupleurum and Poria Formula as a treatment for purpura when conventional medications do not work. It is effective for about twenty percent of patients, comparable to other available treatments for the condition.[4] The formula has been found to be very effective in relieving muscle cramps in patients with liver disease,[5] and helping men maintain normal urination after prostate surgery, although the latter study only involved two patients.[6] More importantly, Bupleurum and Poria Formula has been found useful in treating childhood kidney diseases that are ordinarily treated with steroids, sometimes allowing children to stay off steroid medications for as long as two years.[7]

Interactions with Prescription Drugs

Kampo makers warn that Bupleurum and Poria Formula greatly increases urination in some individuals. It can have a diuretic effect comparable to the prescription drug Lasix (furosemide).

Comparisons to Other Formulas

Minor Bupleurum Decoction by itself may be more effective when there is no swelling anywhere in the body.

Bupleurum Formula to Purify the Liver

This formula is also known as Bupleurum Decoction to Purify the Liver. Purifying the liver refers to ridding the body of the lingering physiological effects of emotional distress.

Japanese Name: Saiko-seikan-to
Chinese Name: Chai Hu Qing Gan Tang
Scientific Name: Formula bupleuri ad purifactionem hepatis

Common Brand Names

Bupleurum & Rehmannia Combination (Lotus Classics, Qualiherb, Sun Ten)
Chai Hu Qing Gan Tang (Lotus Classics, Qualiherb, Sun Ten)
Qing Gan (ProBotanixx)
Saiko-seikan-to (Tsumura*)
(*Made in Japan)

Herbs Used to Make a Single Dose

Bupleurum Root 2.0 g
Scutellaria Root 1.5 g
Phellodendron Bark 1.5 g
Coptis Rhizome 1.5 g
Snake Gourd (Trichosanth) Root 1.5 g
Platycodon Root 1.5 g
Cornelian Cherry Fruit 1.5 g
Rehmannia Root 1.5 g

Peony Root 1.5 g
Cnidium Rhizome 1.5 g
Angelica Root 1.5 g
Mint Leaf and Stems 1.5 g
Forsythia Fruit 1.5 g
Arctium Seed 1.5 g

Health Conditions Treated

Age spots, freckles, eczema and chronic, recurrent laryngitis, sore throat, and tonsillitis.

Who Should Use This Formula?

Anyone who suffers recurrent upper respiratory or middle ear infections. In Japan, this formula is often recommended for children.

Consider This Formula If You Have Any of the Health Conditions Listed Above and Experience

Recurrent inflammation of the upper respiratory system, tendency for chronic disease, area with accumulation of pigment, and/or tenderness below the rib cage on the right side.

Energy Diagnosis

This formula is appropriate for an energy diagnosis of:

- Second Stage of Disease
- Yang deficiency
- Heart and liver in a condition of relative Yang excess causing uprising heat, restlessness, nervousness, and inflammation of lymph nodes along the sides of the throat

Explanation

This formula is one of the relatively "new" herbal preparations of Kampo, only recorded in the Chinese medical text *Golden Mirror of Medical Tradition* in 1742. It treats a variety of conditions in which "toxins" accumulate in the throat and skin causing burning (such as sore throat) or "scorching" (such as age spots, eczema, or freckles). In the energy condition treated by this formula, the emotional energies that are normally contained in the liver escape to the throat and skin. Since the "fire" caused by toxins naturally rises upward, symptoms are more pronounced in the upper parts of the body. Age spots and freckles will occur on the face before they occur on the hands, and severe headache may precede sore throat and laryngitis. Fiery energies may "coalesce" into phlegm and nasal congestion, or they may cause skin inflammation of eczema or herpes, or they may simply cause redness of the face and bad breath.

Many modern authorities consider these herbs to be *the* formula for treating eczema or chronic throat in cases in which the person is under constant emotional stress. It is particularly useful for stopping pain, calming the mind, and relieving the symptoms of inflammation in the throat and skin. It also is thought to ensure the downward flow of energy from the intestines, preventing "sugar highs" and nervousness after meals.

Documentation

There have been no clinical tests of this formula as a whole, and laboratory studies with animals have only confirmed that it has a remarkable ability to stimulate the flow of bile.[1] A study of a closely related formula, Gentiana Longdancao Formula to Drain the Liver, found that the herbs slow down the digestion of proteins from food that may activate eczema and other kinds of skin inflammation.[2]

Some of the effects of the formula may be explained in terms of what is known of its constituent herbs. Bupleurum stops the effects of allergies by blocking 5HT, a substance that makes the walls of capillaries permeable to fluids leaking into soft tissues and causing them to swell, especially the soft tissues lining the nose and throat and lying under the skin.[3] Recent research has found that mint contains 8 chemical compounds that act as antihistamines.[4] Trichosanth root stops allergies, strangely, by providing a large amount of plant-made histamine, to which the body reacts with an anti-inflammatory reaction.[5]

Cinnamon Formula

This formula is also known as Cinnamon Twig Decoction.

Japanese Name: Keishi-to
Chinese Name: Gui Zhi Tang
Scientific Name: Formula cinnamomi

Common Brand Names

Children's Sentinel (Three Treasures)
Cinnamon Combination (Lotus Classics, Qualiherb, Sun Ten)
Cinnamon Twig Formula (Golden Flower Chinese Herbs)
Gui Zhi Tang (Lotus Classics, Qualiherb, Sun Ten)
Kampo4Cold/Flu Cinnamon Formula (Honso*)
Keishi-to (Tsumura*)
(*Made in Japan)

Herbs Used to Make a Single Dose

Cinnamon Bark 4.0 g
Peony Root 4.0 g
Jujube Fruit 4.0 g
Licorice Root 2.0 g
Ginger (fresh) 1.0 g

Health Conditions Treated

Initial stages of bronchitis, colds, flu, sinusitis, and other respiratory infections accompanied by fever and chills.

Consider This Formula If You Have Any of the Health Conditions Listed Above and Experience

Any level of fatigue requiring interruption of normal physical activities, pain around the eyes, stiff muscles in the neck or shoulders, nasal congestion, sweating that does not relieve fever, dry eyes, and/or inability to concentrate. It is also appropriate if you experience a burning sensation anywhere in the digestive tract (heartburn, burning pain of the anus during bowel movement) after taking antibiotics or over-the-counter medications for bronchitis or any upper respiratory infections.

Energy Diagnosis

This formula is appropriate for an energy diagnosis of:

- First Stage of Disease
- *Ki* deficiency

Explanation

Nearly two thousand years ago the master herbalist Zhang Zhong-jing originally designed Cinnamon Formula to treat the first few days of diseases thought to be carried on a cold winter wind. Zhang believed that the unpleasant symptoms of bronchitis, colds, flu, and sinus inflammation were caused not by an infectious microorganism but rather by an imbalance of the body's vital energy, *ki*.

One way *ki* could become unbalanced was by overexertion in the cold. Heavy physical exercise causes sweating. The opening of the pores during sweating makes the person more sensitive to the environment, which leads to sensitivity to cold temperatures and a susceptibility to catching cold. Any other kind of drain on energy could also cause an imbalance of *ki*. In a cold wind, the body directs protective energy to the lungs. When vital energy is drawn away from the stomach to reinforce the lungs, the nutritive energy of the stomach is no longer able to contain fluids. Some of these fluids travel up in the body to cause runny nose. There also could be copious sweating without any effect on fever or diarrhea along with the expected runny nose and chest congestion. The Yang energies taken from the digestive tract rise through all the Yang channels, which meet in the head. There they collide and cause headache, sore throat, and itchy nasal passages.

A damp cold wind could cause the pathogenic process through

which the *ki* becomes misdirected. The pathogenic influence this formula battles is known in Chinese medicine as *feng shui* (with the same meaning as the practice of directing energies in interior design, popularly known as *feng shui*). This condition is a teaming up of the pathogenic influences of Wind and Water. In *feng shui* the lungs are simply unable to process damp air and take in water as well as air. If the body could generate enough protective *qi*, this would not be a problem, but generally there has been a wearing down of the defenses to make this impossible. People who are susceptible to this kind of attack usually had allergies, tonsillitis, or recurrent respiratory infections in their younger years, and their weak respiratory system caused them to refrain from vigorous physical activity.

Since the pathogenic energy of wind is associated with an inability to choose or to distinguish between what is important and what is not, people who have weak lung function as children tend, in the thought of traditional Japanese medicine, to grow into nervous adults. They tend to worry too much about details, and to crave food without really being hungry and without ever feeling really satisfied. They usually prefer sweet foods and food high in liquid content. They tend to belch and release gas, and complain of pain in the shoulders and knees. After decades of duress, the body loses its inner sense of direction with regard to fluids. These people tend to get digestive disturbances when they get colds.

Later Japanese physicians interpreted the expenditure of energy required to make difficult decisions as the same kind of disease influence as a cold wind. Any drain of this kind of energy could lead to a predisposition to bronchitis, colds, sinusitis, and flu. Drinking heavily at a party or celebration, using tranquilizers, or any chronic environmental or personal annoyance had the same effect as a winter wind, as well as the same treatment.

The observations of Kampo physicians have their analogies in modern medicine. At least some strains of the virus that causes the common cold only become infectious when they penetrate the adhesion molecules, the "pores," between the cells lining the nose. At least one study, published in the prestigious *New England Journal of Medicine*, confirms that people under psychological stress are more likely to catch colds.[1] The more elaborate theory of the relationship between upper respiratory infections and emotions, however, remains the exclusive domain of Kampo medicine.

Documentation

Since the herbs of Cinnamon Formula are used as the basis for twenty other formulas, they are exceptionally well researched. Zhang Zhongjing used cinnamon to release the "exterior," or immune system, from the effects of invading cold. The volatile oils in cinnamon are known to be antiviral, antifungal, and antibacterial.[2] Peony was included to help the body contain energies that would "rise to the surface" to cause spontaneous sweating or seating at night. Peony increases the white blood cell count, and has antispasmodic, sedative, analgesic, and fever-lowering properties.[3] Ginger was included in the formula to assist cinnamon in expelling cold. At least forty scientific studies confirm that ginger can counteract digestive disturbance. It contains the compound beta-sesquiphellandrene, which kills cold virus (rhinovirus) at a concentration of less than one part per million (which is approximately its concentration in this formula).[4] Jujube "harmonized" the body's digestive and defensive *ki*. Jujube is an outstanding source of ascorbic acid, the green fruit consisting of 1.0% vitamin C.[5] While jujube is not known to have any effect on the interrelationship between the digestive system and the immune system, it is known to protect the digestive system from toxins. Laboratory tests show that jujube protects the liver from toxins such as carbon tetrachloride.[6] Licorice was thought to harmonize energies. Numerous scientific studies have found that compounds in licorice help the body conserve the inflammation-reducing hormones known as cortisols,[7] which help the body reduce inflammation of the mucous membranes and quell digestive upset.

One of the more interesting studies of the formula as a whole offers some confirmation of its traditional use in relieving the stress of making difficult decisions. Scientists at the International Traditional Medicine

Research Center in Toyama, Japan, tested Cinnamon Formula as a means of changing contingent negative variation, a measurement of brain activity associated with attention, will power, and motivation. They found that subjects taking the formula experienced lower levels of contingent negative variation for a short time after taking the formula, but that their brain activity recovered after less than an hour.[8]

Comparisons to Other Formulas

Cyperus and Perilla Powder may be more effective when common cold or flu has lasted more than a week before beginning treatment, or is accompanied by marked depression or fatigue.

Ginseng Formula may be added to treat runny nose.

Kudzu Decoction may be more effective if stiff muscles in the neck and shoulders are the primary symptom.

Ligusticum and Green Tea Powder will relieve severe headaches associated with colds or flu.

Cinnamon, Dragon Bone, and Oyster Shell Formula

Many reference books refer to this formula as Cinnamon Twig Decoction plus Dragon Bone and Oyster Shell. "Dragon bone" refers to pulverized fossil bones, commonly used as a calming agent in Kampo medicine.

Japanese Name: Keishi-ka-ryukotsu-borei-to
Chinese Name: Gui Zhi Jia Long Gu Mu Li Tang
Scientific Name: Formula cinnamomi cum ostrea et fossilia ossis

Common Brand Names

Cinnamon & D.B. Combination (Sun Ten)
Cinnamon & Dragon Bone Combination (Lotus Classics)

Cinnamon & Peony (Qualiherb)
Cinnamon and Dragon Bone (Qualiherb)
Cinnamon D Formula (Golden Flower Chinese Herbs)
Cinnamon Twig Plus (Alembic Herbals)
Gui Zhi Jia Long Mu Li Tang (Alembic Herbals, Golden Flower Chinese Herbs, Lotus Classics, Qualiherb, Sun Ten)
Keishi-ka-ryukotsu-borei-to (Tsumura*)
(*Made in Japan)

Herbs Used to Make a Single Dose

Cinnamon Bark 4.0 g
Peony Root 4.0 g
Jujube Fruit 4.0 g
Oyster Shell 3.0 g
Dragon Bone 3.0 g
Licorice Root 2.0 g
Ginger (fresh) 1.5 g

Some Japanese-made formulations of this product substitute inorganic sources of calcium for oyster shell and dragon bone to meet kosher requirements.

Health Conditions Treated

Pain after vasectomy, erectile dysfunction, varicocele, excessive urination, insomnia, migraine, and nightmares.

Who Should Use This Formula?

Physically weakened patients, especially those suffering poor nutrition.

Consider This Formula If You Have Any of the Health Conditions

Listed Above and Experience

Exhaustion or easy fatigue after exercise, nightsweats, cold hands and feet, and/or excessive urination of clear urine. In men: loss of interest in sex and/or erectile dysfunction.

Energy Diagnosis

This formula is appropriate for an energy diagnosis of:

- Second Stage of Disease
- Yin deficiency in the kidneys. Shallow sleep with abundant dreams is a sign of weakness of the heart.

Explanation

The students of Zhang Zhong-jing devised this formula in the late third century A.D. to treat sexual dysfunctions in both men and women. These ancient Chinese physicians saw sexual dysfunction primarily as a communication problem, that is, a failure of the kidneys and the heart to communicate *ki* to one another. In the thinking of third-century Kampo, excessive sexual activity, whether physical or mental (that is, thinking about or dreaming about sex), depleted the kidneys of their energy essence. The kidneys lost their ability to contain the *ki* energy that makes Yang (outwardly directed) activity possible. This Yang drifted up to the heart, where it disturbed dreams, rather than down to the sex organs, to enable erections in men and orgasms in women. Yin energies accumulate in the sex organs and cause coldness, which may be literal—that is, a cold sensation in the genitals—or figurative, an inability to respond to stimulation. As Yang energies continue to flow upward away from the reproductive organs, there may be dizziness, palpitations, insomnia, and dream-disturbed sleep. In men, upward-flowing Yang causes hair loss.

In twenty-first century Chinese herbal medicine, this formula is used to treat fatigue from overwork or excessive sexual activity *before* there are symptoms of sexual dysfunction. It is also recommended to patients who present lower back pain or coldness in the extremities.

Documentation

On a molecular level, Cinnamon, Dragon Bone, and Oyster Shell Formula complements the pharmacological action of Viagra. (This formula will *not* enable erection in men after a single administration.) Viagra *increases* the production of free radicals of nitric oxide (NO). These enhance circulation to the sex organs in both men and women. The "dragon bone" and oyster shell component of Cinnamon, Dragon Bone, and Oyster Shell formula *decreases* the production of other free radicals, specifically the superoxide radical and hydroxyl radical, which cause the vascular damage for which Viagra compensates.[1]

Clear Summerheat and Augment the Qi Formula

In traditional East Asian medicine, summerheat is an environmental insult that causes "diseases that are not quite diseases." Exposure to summer's heat and humidity, or deprivation of air and sunshine inside air-conditioned homes and offices, gradually depletes the body of vital *ki* and sets the stage for disease. This formula clears summer's heat from the body and boosts *ki* to prevent disease.

Japanese Name: Seisho-ekki-to
Chinese Name: Qing Shu Yi Qi Tang
Scientific Name: Formula ad auxilium vis vitalis et contra refrigerationem

Common Brands

- Astragalus & Atractylodis (Qualiherb)
- Astragalus & Atractylodis Combination (Lotus Classics, Sun Ten)
- Qing Shu (Alembic Herbals)
- Qing Shu Yi Qi Tang (Alembic Herbals, Lotus Classics, Qualiherb, Sun Ten)

Seisho-ekki-to (Tsumura*)
(*Made in Japan)

Herbs Used to Make a Single Dose

White Atractylodis Rhizome 3.5 g
Ginseng 3.5 g
Sprouted Barley Seed 3.5 g
Astragalus Root 3.0 g
Chen-Pi Peel 3.0 g
Angelica Root 3.0 g
Phellodendron Bark 1.0 g
Licorice Root 1.0 g
Schisandra Fruit 1.0 g

Health Conditions Treated

Heat stress and hyperthyroidism.

Who Should Use This Formula?

People whose daily routine has been interrupted by heat stress.

Consider This Formula If You Have Any of the Health Conditions Listed Above and Experience

Fatigue due to summer heat, loss of appetite, loose stools, scanty urination, sweating, and/or hot hands and feet.

Energy Diagnosis

This formula is appropriate for an energy diagnosis of:

- Second Stage of Disease
- Yang deficiency
- *Ki* deficiency. Disease resistance is weak and diseases contracted in this state tend to become chronic.

Explanation

This formula is a relatively recent addition to the repertoire of Japanese Kampo. It was first documented in a Chinese medical text entitled *The Warp and Woof of Warm-Febrile Diseases* in 1852, although it may have been devised by a doctor Ye Tian Shi in the late seventeenth century. During this period in the development of Kampo medicine, physicians sought a more concise way of describing the Six Stages of Disease. They noted that heat stress, in particular, seemed to move through four different kinds of energies in the body.

The first energy level disturbed by the heat of summer is the immune system. Fighting heat makes it difficult for the body to fight infection. Only after the heat of summer has overcome the immune system, Kampo physicians reasoned, does it begin to sap the body's vital energy. The *ki* that roughly corresponds to "get up and go" is lost when summer heat disrupts this second energy layer. Heat stress goes on to interfere with the digestion of food at the third level of *ki* and finally with the blood itself. The fourth and final stage of heat stress at the level of the blood can cause drastic fluctuations in the fluid content of the body. Fluids are sweated out so profusely that the blood becomes "viscous." Merely drinking water is not enough to make blood "slippery" again. It is also necessary to augment the *ki* so that blood and fluids resume their normal flow throughout the body.

Documentation

While there has only been a single preliminary scientific study of this formula's effectiveness, the research was carefully planned as a test of the formula's ability to treat the conditions described in the original texts. Scientists at the Product Development Laboratories of Lion Corporation in Kanagawa, Japan, first measured the effects of housing laboratory animals at a temperature of 34° C (93° F) in high humidity for three days and nights. The scientists made sure food and water were freely available to the animals in the test. They found that over the seventy-two-hour period the animals' blood volume decreased as fluids moved out of the bloodstream and into the surrounding tissues.

Researchers concluded that this condition matched the *suitai* syndrome described in nineteenth-century medical books.

Then the scientists gave the test animals Clear Summerheat and Augment the *Qi* Formula once a day for five days. The herbal formula reversed the distribution of body fluids induced by high temperature. It enabled the kidneys to operate more efficiently in handling increased water consumption triggered by high temperatures.[1] Fluids moved out of the tissues and into the bloodstream, from which they could be eliminated by the kidneys. Subsequent weakness and infection associated with the *suitai* syndrome did not occur.

Comparisons to Other Formulas

Ten-Significant Tonic Decoction may be more effective when there is profuse sweating but no diarrhea.

Tonify the Middle and Augment the *Qi* Formula may be more effective when there is only mild sweating and no diarrhea.

Coptis Antidote

This formula is also widely known as Coptis Decoction to Relieve Toxicity.

Japanese Name: Oren-gedoku-to
Chinese Name: Huang Lian Jie Du Tang
Scientific Name: Formula coptidis et antidoti

Common Brand Names

CoptiDetox (Kan Traditionals)
Coptis & Scute Combination (Lotus Classics, Sun Ten)
Coptis & Scute Formula (Chinese Classics)

Coptis & Scutellaria (Qualiherb)
Huang Lian Jie Du Tang (Chinese Classics, Kan Traditionals, Lotus Classics, Qualiherb, Sun Ten)
Oregedokuto Formula 016 (Kampo Institute*)
Oren-gedoku-to (Honso,* Tsumura*)
(* Made in Japan)

Herbs Used to Make a Single Dose

Scutellaria Root 3.0 g
Coptis Rhizome 2.0 g
Gardenia Fruit 2.0 g
Phellodendron Bark 1.5 g

Health Conditions Treated

Depression, dysmenorrhea, hypertension, nosebleed, tachycardia (racing pulse), vertigo, and any condition in which there is vomiting or coughing of blood. In Japan, this formula is widely used in the long-term care of stroke patients.

Who Should Use This Formula?

Physically active individuals whose daily activities are not limited by disease.

Consider This Formula If You Have Any of the Health Conditions Listed Above and Experience

"Red" symptoms, such as bleeding, fever, redness in the face, rashes, etc.

Energy Diagnosis

This formula is appropriate for an energy diagnosis of:

- Second Stage of Disease
- Yang deficiency
- *Ki* stasis
- *Oketsu*

Explanation

Coptis Antidote was brought to Japanese herbal medicine via an eighth-century Chinese medical text entitled *Arcane Essentials from the Imperial Library*. The physicians of the time used this combination of herbs to treat "fire toxins" that overwhelmed the triple burners, an energy organ of Traditional Chinese Medicine roughly corresponding to the immune system. The potent herbs of this formula were required when the inflammatory toxins caused by infections or severe disturbances of *ki* had overwhelmed not only the exterior energy layers of the body but the interior energy layers of the body as well.

What conditions create a fire toxin? While most practitioners readily identify fire toxins associated with inflammatory infections, modern Kampo physician Giovanni Maciocia theorizes that anger, frustration, and resentment become energetically "fiery" over time. Combined with overwork or excessive sexual activity, these energies begin to poison the immune system with physical, mental, and even spiritual results. Persons suffering from fire toxins of the triple burners lose their sense of direction in life and become depressed. Since the energies of the liver can no longer house what Chinese Kampo medicine calls the Ethereal Soul, sleep becomes disturbed and nightmares proliferate. In extreme cases, there may be symptoms Western medicine associates with the manic phase of bipolar disorder.

Documentation

While no scientific study documents the effects of Coptis Antidote on the Ethereal Soul, there have been no fewer than forty-two scientific studies of various pharmacological effects of the formula as a whole and no fewer than eighty-seven studies of its principal herb, coptis. Many of the formulas used in Kampo are only documented in research journals published in Chinese or Japanese, but the most recent studies of Coptis Antidote have been published in English in mainstream pharmacological journals printed in the United States.

Among the earlier scientific studies of Coptis Antidote was a

Japanese experiment designed to evaluate the efficacy of the formula in treating gastric bleeding. Tests with laboratory animals found that Coptis Antidote stopped bleeding induced by alcohol or aspirin.[1] The next round of research tested the traditional application of Coptis Antidote as a treatment for stroke patients. Japanese physicians frequently describe stroke as an especially severe form of *oketsu*. A clinical study of twenty *oketsu* patients (who had a medical diagnosis of stroke) and twenty healthy volunteers found that the formula slowed the rate at which blood clots form. Moreover, this blood-thinning effect was more pronounced in stroke patients than in the volunteers.[2] Subsequent studies of the formula found that it slowed the rate at which free radicals of oxygen attacked the cholesterol-rich linings of brain cells when flow of oxygenated blood was restored to them after stroke.[3] Yet another team of investigators found that Coptis Antidote preserved the linings of human liver cells exposed to toxic chemicals.[4]

All of the studies of Coptis Antidote published since 1999 have been conducted in the laboratory without human subjects. Scientists at Tsumura & Company found that the chemical berberine, released by the herbs in the formula when they are prepared as a tea (or prepared as a tea for concentration into tablet form), slows the rate at which immune-protective T-cells progress through their normal life cycle. Berberine increases the time T-cells are available to fight disease.[5] In other studies using animals to model human diseases, Coptis Antidote prevents death of brain tissue during oxygen deprivation,[6] suppresses the formation of pre-cancerous lesions of the colon,[7] inhibits the allergic reactions that cause dermatitis,[8] complements standard treatments for colitis and Crohn's disease,[9] and reduces the risk of impairment of learning and memory after stroke.[10]

Note: When using any formula containing coptis, it is important to take no more than the recommended dosage. Small amounts of coptis stimulate the brain and result in alertness, while large amounts induce drowsiness. Similarly, small doses of coptis increase blood pressure, but large doses of coptis lower it.

Dong Quai and Gentian Formula

This formula is also known as Gentiana Longdancao Decoction to Drain the Liver. "Draining the liver" refers to removing the physiological effects of fiery emotions.

Japanese Name: Ryutan-shakan-to
Chinese Name: Long Dan Xie Gan Tang
Scientific Name: Formula pacificationis hepatis gentianae scabrae

Common Brand Names

Drain Fire (Three Treasures)
Gentiana Combination (Lotus Classics)
Gentiana Drain Fire Formula (Golden Flower Chinese Herbs)
Gentiana Formula (Chinese Classics)
Long Dan Xie Gan Tang (Chinese Classics, Golden Flower Chinese Herbs, Health Concerns, Jade Pharmacy, Kan Herbals, Lotus Classics, ProBotanixx, Three Treasures)
Quell Fire (Jade Pharmacy, Kan Herbals)
Ryutan-shakan-to (Honso,* Tsumura*)
Yi Jun (ProBotanixx)
(* Made in Japan)

Herbs Used to Make a Single Dose

Rehmannia Root 5.0 g
Angelica Root 5.0 g
Akebia Caulis 5.0 g
Scutellaria Root 5.0 g
Psyllium Seed 3.0 g
Alisma Rhizome 3.0 g

Licorice Root 1.0 g
Gardenia Fruit 1.0 g
Gentian Root 1.0 g

Health Conditions Treated

Pelvic inflammatory disease, vaginitis, and yeast infections.

Who Should Use This Formula?

Women with a tendency for weight gain who suffer acute or chronic inflammation of the urogenital tract.

Consider This Formula If You Have Any of the Health Conditions Listed Above and Experience

Inflammation of the urinary tract, feeling of incomplete urination, scanty urination, turbid urine, white discharge from the vagina, and/or a feeling of heat throughout the body.

Energy Diagnosis

This formula is appropriate for an energy diagnosis of:

- Third Stage of Disease
- Yang Symptoms
- *Ki* neither excessive nor deficient
- Stasis of fluids

Explanation

Dong Quai and Gentian Formula was recorded by the Chinese physician Wang Ang in 1682. It is one of several formulas that use gentian primarily to treat women's conditions. Gentian is the herb of choice in Kampo medicine for conditions caused by fire. This misplaced emotional energy begins as anger, frustration, or overwork. Over a period of months or years it can overcome the energies of immune defenses and begun to sap vital *ki*, causing fatigue and constant risk of infection.

Kampo physicians recognize the syndrome for which this formula is most helpful as a manifestation of fiery energies in female patients. Fire causes red symptoms. When this formula is appropriate, there is usually redness of the face or tongue. Fire dries up fluids. In the symptom pattern for which this formula is especially useful there may be dry mouth, a lingering bitter taste after eating, and reduced volume of urination. Flames rise upward. This formula treats headache, tendency to explosive temper, and ill-considered or manic behavior. Flames scorch. Women who benefit from Dong Quai and Gentian Formula tend to suffer constipation and their urine will be dark. Finally, fire carries particles aloft. The *Yellow Emperor's Classic of Internal Medicine* notes that "All that rebels and rushes upward is associated with fire; vomiting and acid regurgitation are associated with heat." In the symptom pattern relieved by this herbal treatment, there may be vomiting, belching, or acid reflux.

Many modern practitioners of Kampo medicine caution against the use of the formula to treat "heat" rather than "fire." This formula is highly effective, but may be too strong for mild symptoms.

Documentation

Physicians at the Osaka Prefectural Institute of Public Health in Japan have attempted to ascertain the mechanism through which Dong Quai and Gentian Formula controls gastrointestinal symptoms. Their initial investigations have found that the formula greatly reduces the stomach's release of the digestive enzyme pancreatin.[1] This action slows down the digestive process so that there is a lesser flow of stomach acids and reduced vomiting, belching, and acid reflux.

Comparisons to Other Formulas

Five-Ingredient Powder for Painful Urinary Dysfunction may be more effective for especially severe inflammation of the urinary tract.

Lotus Seed Formula to Clear the Kidneys may bolster Dong Quai and Gentian Formula's infection-fighting effects.

Polyporus Formula should be taken in addition to Dong Quai and Gentian Formula when there is failure to urinate and sore throat.

Dong Quai and Peony Formula

This combination of herbs is also known as Tang-kuei and Peony Formula.

Japanese Name: Toki-shakuyaku-san
Chinese Name: Dan Gui Shao Yao San
Scientific Name: Pulvis paeoniae et angelicae

Common Brand Names

Dang Gui & Peony (Qualiherb)
Kampo4Women MenopauEase (Honso*)
Tangkuei & Peony Formula (Lotus Classics)
Tang-Kuei and Peony Formula (Golden Flower Chinese Herbs, Sun Ten)
Toki-shakuyaku-san (Honso,* Tsumura*)
(* Made in Japan)

Herbs Used to Make a Single Dose

Peony Root 4.0 g
White Atractylodis Root 4.0 g
Alisma Rhizome 4.0 g
Angelica Root 3.0 g
Poria 4.0 g
Ligusticum Root 3.0 g

Health Conditions Treated

Alzheimer's disease, discomforts of menopause, and menstrual irregularity.

Who Should Use This Formula?

Women whose health conditions interfere with their lifestyle choices.

Consider This Formula If You Have Any of the Health Conditions Listed Above and Experience

Fatigue; anemia; sensitivity to cold; swelling before, during, and after menstruation; abdominal pain; headache; stiff neck and shoulders; racing pulse; abdominal pain; and/or hemorrhoids.

Energy Diagnosis

This formula is appropriate for an energy diagnosis of:

- Fourth Stage of Disease
- Yin excess
- *Ki* deficiency
- Oketsu

Explanation

Dong Quai and Peony Formula is the East Asian equivalent of black cohosh. Practitioners of Traditional Chinese Medicine use this formula to treat abnormalities of the "girdle vessel." This is an energy channel that keeps *ki* from becoming "slack" and sinking too low in the body.

The mechanism through which this formula stiffens up the flow of *ki* is by "nourishing the liver." Increasing the supply of *ki* to the liver prevents symptoms wherever the liver's energies flow in the body. Correcting liver energy problems corrects poor memory, insomnia, blurred vision, dry eyes, dry hair, broken nails, and/or tingling sensations in the hands or feet associated with any of the medical conditions for which this formula is indicated.

Documentation

Physicians in Japan prescribe Dong Quai and Peony Powder to treat a wide range of women's health concerns. These are conditions that American physicians frequently ignore, or for which they recommend surgery or harsh pharmaceutical preparations that remove estrogen from circulation.[1] In women who have not yet reached menopause, Dong Quai and Peony formula increases the production of estrogen when it is needed but not when it could cause premenstrual syndrome. During the first fourteen days of the menstrual cycle, the formula stimulates ovulation and stops outbreaks of acne by causing the ovaries to produce more estrogen and less testosterone.

In women who have reached menopause and women who take drugs that reduce the availability of estrogen (usually to treat breast cancer, endometriosis, fibrocystic breast disease, and uterine fibroids), the formula relieves side effects of medication, such as hot flashes, nausea, vomiting, and shoulder pain. It does this without increasing estrogen levels.[2] The formula regulates estrogen without disturbing its delicate balance with testosterone,[3] preserving sex drive and preventing "masculinizing" side effects.

When estrogen is in balance with testosterone, abnormal hair growth and disturbances of libido are relatively rare. In the case of endometriosis, Dong Quai and Peony Powder reduces the formation of inflammatory compounds in endometrial tissue.[4] While the formula does not "dissolve" endometrial tissue, it greatly reduces the pain women who have endometriosis experience during the first fourteen days of their period.

Dr. Nobuyoshi Hagino, of Japan's Dokkyo School of Medicine and University of Texas Health Science Center at San Antonio, has been testing Dong Quai and Peony Formula in the treatment of age-related mental decline. Dr. Hagino was among the clinical researchers who discovered that estrogen therapy eases symptoms in women who have Alzheimer's disease. Women with mild Alzheimer's who were given conjugated equine estrogens (drugs like Premarin) regained some ability to function in daily life and to communicate with family and friends. Since Dong Quai and Peony Formula helps women's bodies preserve estrogen, Dr. Hagino wondered whether it might have a beneficial effect on Alzheimer's Disease.

Dr. Hagino's research team found that Kampo medicine was even more effective than estrogen. Women given this Japanese herbal formula not only recovered social skills, they showed significant improvement in conversation, reading, and writing, and in both short- and long-term memory.[5] The women in the pilot study began to pay attention to dress and makeup. Unlike conjugated equine estrogens, Dong Quai and Peony Formula caused no side effects.

Comparisons to Other Formulas

Dong Quai and Peach Seed Formula may be a helpful addition to Dong Quai and Peony Formula when there are bleeding hemorrhoids or areas of dark pigmentation on the skin, such as age spots or freckles.

Major Ledebouriella Formula may be taken simultaneously with Dong Quai and Peony Formula when there is also muscle atrophy or weakness, or arthritis.

Eight-Ingredient Pill with Rehmannia

Many practitioners of Traditional Chinese Medicine refer to this herbal combination as Rehmannia Eight Formula.

Japanese Name: Hachimi-jio-gan
Chinese Name: Ba Wei Di Huang Wan
Scientific Name: Formula rehmanniae et octo-medicamentorum

Common Brand Names

Ba Wei Di Huang Wan (Health Concerns, Honso,* Lotus Classics, Qualiherb, Sun Ten)
Hachimi-jio-gan (Tsumura*)
Hachimijiogan Formula 019 (Kampo Institute*)

Prostate Kampo (Honso*)
Rehmannia 8 (Qualiherb)
Rehmannia Eight Formula (Lotus Classics, Sun Ten)
(* Made in Japan)

<u>Herbs Used to Make a Single Dose</u>

Rehmannia Root 6.0 g
Cornelian Cherry Fruit 3.0 g
Dioscorea Root 3.0 g
Alisma Rhizome 3.0 g
Poria 3.0 g
Moutan Root 2.5 g
Cinnamon Bark 1.0 g
Aconite Tuber 0.5 g

<u>Health Conditions Treated</u>

Diabetes, erectile dysfunction, and prostate problems.

<u>Who Should Use This Formula?</u>

Men who are "out of shape" and have been given a medical diagnosis of one of the health conditions listed above.

<u>Consider This Formula If You Have Any of the Health Conditions Listed Above and Experience</u>

Fatigue, either excessive or scanty urination, impotence, pelvic pain, thirst, cold hands and feet, and/or a tendency to develop edema anywhere in the body. Scrotal edema and swollen testicles are especially strong indications for the use of this formula.

<u>Energy Diagnosis</u>

This formula is appropriate for an energy diagnosis of:

- Fourth Stage of Disease
- Yin excess
- Yang deficiency, especially in kidneys

- *Ki* deficiency
- Stasis of fluids

Explanation

Although this formula came to Japanese medicine from a Chinese medical textbook entitled *Women's Diseases According to Fu Qing Zhu*, today it is Kampo's most frequently recommended formula in the treatment of erectile dysfunction, prostate problems, and diabetes in men.

The herbs in the formula are chosen to relieve "bitterness." On a physical level, bitterness refers to the inability of the kidneys and liver to contain Yin fluids. As the kidneys lose their ability to contain fluids, the fluids remaining in them become increasingly concentrated or "bitter."

On a psychological level, bitterness refers to the difficulty of dealing with ongoing emotional tension. This is particularly important if the source of the emotional tension is guilt. Traditional East Asian medicine teaches that guilt harbored for many years damages the kidneys so that dizziness, tinnitus, backache, nightsweats, dry mouth, and exhaustion result.

Documentation

Japanese physicians prescribe Eight-Ingredient Pill with Rehmannia more often than any other herbal formula for diabetes. This formula is useful for both type 1 and type 2 diabetes. It is helpful for diabetics who take insulin and for diabetics who do not. Like other formulas containing the herb rehmannia, it lowers blood sugars, enables the body to use insulin more effectively, and slows and sometimes reverses the progress of diabetic neuropathy. For treating diabetes itself, Eight-Ingredient Pill with Rehmannia is prescribed to men and women.

The primary benefit of Eight-Ingredient Pill with Rehmannia for insulin-dependent diabetics lies in making it easier to maintain "tight control." The formula does not reduce insulin requirements. Instead, it stops blood sugar levels from going up after meals. Keeping blood sugar levels relatively constant is a well-known method for preventing diabetic retinopathy and other problems of blood circulation.[1] The formula has a lesser but significant utility in keeping sugar levels stable in diabetics who do not have to take insulin.

This formula counteracts several common eye problems in people with diabetes. Recent research shows that Eight-Ingredient Pill with Rehmannia brakes a series of inflammatory reactions, mediated by the immune system, that affect nerve tissues. Slowing down the production of Tumor Necrosis Factor preserves both the retina and the optic nerve.

The benefit of Eight-Ingredient Pill with Rehmannia in maintaining sight in diabetes is the prevention of cataracts through inhibition of the enzyme aldose reductase.[2] This enzyme induces a transformation of sugars in the lens of the eye into a form that is stored in microscopic vacuoles, or sacs. These tiny pockets of "gummy" sugars eventually cloud the lens. When aldose reductase is deactivated, galactose sugars cannot accumulate in a harmful form in the lens.

Additionally, this formula helps maintain the balance of sodium, potassium, and calcium in the lens. Electrolyte balance enables a normal flow of fluids in and out of the lens. The "cleansing action" of normal fluid flow helps keep the lens transparent. Normal fluid flow also slows the formation of deposits catalyzed by aldose reductase.[3] Laboratory tests of Eight-Ingredient Pill with Rehmannia in animals suggest that it can delay the development of cataracts by ten to fifteen years in humans.

The usefulness of Eight-Ingredient Pill with Rehmannia in treating erectile dysfunction can be inferred from its usefulness in treating circulatory problems related to diabetes. Like retinopathy, diabetes-related erectile dysfunction occurs when the microvasculature of the penis becomes "clogged." Maintaining blood flow to and within the penis makes erection possible.

Directly relevant laboratory research confirms the use of this formula in treating prostate conditions. Studies indicate that the formula eases urination by altering the thymidine kinase enzyme pathway.[4] When this enzyme is disabled, the amount of testosterone in circulation to the brain to stimulate sex drive increases, but it does not stimulate growth of already enlarged prostate tissues.

Comparisons to Other Formulas

Angelica Formula may be more effective when insomnia and/or depression are present as principal symptoms.

Cinnamon and Oyster Shell Formula may be more effective when there are palpitations, restlessness, fear, or insomnia, and there is *ki* deficiency or imbalance.

Six-Ingredient Pill with Rehmannia may be more effective when there are dry skin outbreaks.

Ephedra Formula

Japanese Name: Mao-to
Chinese Name: Ma Huang Tang
Scientific Name: Formula ephedrae

Common Brand Names

Mahuang Combination (Lotus Classics, Qualiherb, Sun Ten)
Mao-to (Honso,* Tsumura*)
(* Made in Japan)

Herbs Used to Make a Single Dose

Peach Seed 5.0 g
Ephedra Leaf 5.0 g
Cinnamon Bark 4.0 g
Licorice Root 1.5 g

Health Conditions Treated

Bronchitis, colds, flu, and blocked nose in infants.

Who Should Use This Formula?

Physically active individuals who have infectious diseases in the acute stage, infants who have breathing problems when feeding.

Consider This Formula If You Have Any of the Health Conditions Listed Above and Experience

Chills, fever, headache, or nasal congestion, without unusual perspiration.

Energy Diagnosis

This formula is appropriate for an energy diagnosis of:

- First Stage of Disease
- Yang excess causing congestion in the outer layers of the body

Explanation

Most modern practitioners of Kampo medicine consider Ephedra Formula to be the single most effective combination of herbs to treat upper respiratory infections. The energy dynamic of upper respiratory infection is that of an invading cold that has managed to "capture" the immune system's *ki*. Yang energies cannot flow to the exterior of the body, so there are chills. The energy channels carrying Yang converge in the head, so the collision of Yang energies in them results in headache. The lungs cannot transmit their Yang energy upward, so pulmonary energy is expended in wheezing.

Kampo physicians counsel that it is important to remember that this formula is used to treat "Wind-Cold" rather than "Wind-Heat." While the pathogenic energies treated by this formula "come in on a wind," they sap the body's energy rather than activating it. To understand this distinction, consider a colds virus, an allergen, or a sinus infection. These pathogens may be airborne. They do not cause fever, so they may be treated with Ephedra Formula. In contrast, a severe asthma attack (rather than just a mild case of wheezing) causes the body to expend a great deal of energy in tightening breathing passages. Flu causes fever. Asthma and flu are more effectively treated by other formulas. Side effects from the use of ephedra are rare when the appropriate formula is taken.

Documentation

Ephedra is an extraordinarily useful and widely misunderstood herb. The herb ephedra is frequently confused with its best-known pharmacologically active constituent, ephedrine. Although ephedra releases ephedrine and acts through the presence of ephedrine, it also contains many other phytochemicals that buffer and modify ephedrine's effects. Ephedra is generally safe, whereas using ephedrine by itself poses risks of elevated blood pressure and excessive stimulation of the central nervous system. Chemicals in ephedra known as mahuannines, feruloylhistamines, and ephedradines, which are never mentioned in popular literature concerning the risks of using the herb, lower blood pressure and reduce the reactivity of certain parts of the nervous system.

Most of the relief of symptoms by Ephedra Formula is attributable to the release of ephedrine. Shortly after consumption of the herbs, ephedrine enters the bloodstream and crosses the blood-brain barrier. Once inside the brain, it increases the activity of the brain centers that control breathing and blood-vessel contraction. Elsewhere in the body, ephedrine acts a lot like a shot of adrenaline. It triggers the release of chemicals from the ends of nerve fibers in the lungs. These chemicals turn into adrenaline. The flow of adrenaline into the nerves that control the lungs opens breathing passages. The surge of adrenaline helps the heart pump blood more vigorously. This combination of effects allows the formula to relieve symptoms associated with respiratory disorders.

Cinnamon, peach seed, and licorice round out the healing effects of the formula and prevent side effects. Cinnamon contains chemical compounds that block the prostaglandin thromboxane A.[1] This is a hormone that causes blood platelets to clump together, literally clogging arteries and increasing blood pressure. By blocking the prostaglandin, cinnamon dilates the blood vessels and prevents any catastrophic increases in blood pressure. Other compounds in cinnamon are antibacterial, dealing with the infection itself. Peach seeds have their own anticoagulant action in the bloodstream, further lowering the risk of cardiovascular problems that might be caused by overdosing the formula. Licorice prevents digestive upset that might be caused by excessive stimulation of the digestive tract. It reduces inflammation and irritation caused by infection. And while cinnamon is antibacterial, licorice is antiviral, counteracting the other class of microorganisms that causes upper respiratory infection.

Research shows that Ephedra Decoction not only treats the symptoms of colds but can prevent the spread of colds when used at the earliest stages of infection. It is also useful in treating body aches caused by rheumatoid arthritis. Other clinical research has also found that the formula can prevent skin injury from ultraviolet radiation.[2, 3]

Comparisons to Other Formulas

Kudzu Formula may be more effective when there is pain in the neck or back not due to arthritis, in addition to the symptoms usually treated with Ephedra Formula.

Note: Because of the buffering herbs in this formula, it is not likely to cause the side effects that might occur from taking ephedra or ephedrine tablets by themselves. Even so, this formula should not be used for more than two weeks at a time, and it is important to drink eight glasses of water a day while taking this formula to avoid dehydration.

Frigid Extremities Powder

Japanese Name: Shigyaku-san
Chinese Name: Si Ni San
Scientific Name: Pulvis quadrorum medicamentorum

Common Brand Names

Bupleurum & Chih-shih Formula (Lotus Classics, Sun Ten)
Bupleurum & Aurantium (Qualiherb)
Si Ni San (Lotus Classics, Qualiherb, Sun Ten)
Shigyaku-san (Honso,* Tsumura*)
(* Made in Japan)

Herbs Used to Make a Single Dose

Bupleurum Root 5.0 g
Peony Root 4.0 g
Licorice Root 3.0 g
Bitter Orange (Whole) 1.0 g

Health Conditions Treated

Acid reflux, bronchitis, gallbladder irritation, gallstones, gastric ulcer, and nasal allergies.

Who Should Use This Formula?

Physically active persons whose lifestyles are not compromised by disease.

Consider This Formula If You Have Any of the Health Conditions Listed Above and Experience

Tension in the abdominal muscles, mood swings, insomnia, palpitations, bloating, gas, and/or sweaty palms and feet.

Energy Diagnosis

This formula is appropriate for an energy diagnosis of:

- Second Stage of Disease
- *Ki* neither deficient nor excessive.
- Yang deficiency

Explanation

The first generation of the students of Zhang Zhong-jing devised this formula for a peculiar combination of symptoms in which *ki* was simultaneously deficient and excessive in different organs but neither deficient nor excessive in the body as a whole. In modern terms, this formula treats a condition in which the body is "wound up" from emotional distress.

In addition to stress, a congenitally weak constitution, overwork, overexertion, excessive sexual activity, irregular eating habits, childbirth, severe illness, and abuse of alcohol and drugs can cause the liver to become "congested" with emotions. Congested *ki* in the liver deprives the digestive process of the energy it needs for normal activity. There may be belching, vomiting, or diarrhea, and there is almost always a loss of appetite. (As first discussed in Chapter 2, loss of appetite does not always mean eating less food. Loss of appetite may refer to eating greater amounts of food of lesser nutritive value.)

The frigid extremities to which the name of the formula refers are a symptom this particular energy imbalance. The "spleen," or digestive function, provides energy to the flesh. The farther the organ is from the digestive tract, the less energy reaches it. Therefore, when the digestive function is impaired by its own failure to receive energy, the hands and feet will be cold.

Documentation

The single study of this formula involving human volunteers found that it stimulates circulation without stimulating the central nervous system. This distinguishes it from herbal formulas containing ephedra. Japanese pharmacologists classify this formula as a parasympathomimetic.[1] That is, it increases secretions throughout the body, increases the tone of the smooth muscles lining blood vessels, and slows the heart rate.

Comparisons to Other Formulas

Bupleurum, Dragon Bone, and Oyster Shell Formula offers more effective relief of emotional symptoms and may be combined with this formula.

Ginseng Formula to Nourish the Nutritive Qi

The name of this formula refers to a condition in which disease has overcome two of four levels of the body's *ki* (in Chinese, *qi*). It has defeated the first energy level, the immune system, and the second level, at which it has induced fatigue. Now it is interfering with the normal function of the body's third energy level, the nutritive *ki*, corresponding to the body's ability to process nutrients. The herbs in this formula are designed to help restore normal digestive function during chronic disease.

Japanese Name: Ninjin-yoei-to
Chinese Name: Ren Shen Yang Ying Tang
Scientific Name: Formula ginseng compositae

Common Brand Names

Ginseng & Rehmannia Combination (Lotus Classics)
Ginseng Nutritive Formula (Chinese Classics)
Ninjin-yoei-to (Honso,* Tsumura*)
Ren Shen Yang Ying Tang (Chinese Classics, Lotus Classics)
(* Made in Japan)

Herbs Used to Make a Single Dose

Rehmannia Root 4.0 g
Angelica Root 4.0 g
Wild Angelica Root 4.0 g
Poria 4.0 g
Ginseng 3.0 g
Cinnamon 2.5 g

Polygala Root 2.0 g
Peony Root 2.0 g
Chen-Pi Peel 2.0 g
Astragalus Root 1.5 g
Licorice Root 1.0 g
Schisandra Fruit 1.0 g

Health Conditions Treated

Chronic asthma, chronic bronchitis, emphysema, and tuberculosis.

Who Should Use This Formula?

Persons who have chronic breathing problems.

Consider This Formula If You Have Any of the Health Conditions Listed Above and Experience

Exhaustion, cough, palpitations, nightsweats, forgetfulness, cough, dry skin, dry mouth, and/or dry throat.

Energy Diagnosis

This formula is appropriate for an energy diagnosis of:

- Fourth Stage of Disease
- Yin excess
- Systemic *ki* deficiency but relative Yang excess in lung and heart shown as racing pulse, cough, and tendency to fever.

Explanation

This formula treats a condition ancient Kampo medicine identified as "chest painful obstruction syndrome." This energy imbalance is characterized by a feeling of oppression and pain in the chest. The pain may extend to the shoulders. In most cases, "oppression" is a more significant symptom than pain, but in some cases there may be a stabbing pain in the area of the heart.

Zhang Zhong-jing taught that the seven emotions (happiness, anger, worry, pensiveness, grief, fear, and surprise) and the six energy evils (pathogenic wind, cold, wetness, dryness, summerheat, and heat) aggravated a condition of painful obstruction in the chest. His basic idea was that worry, brooding, and pensiveness burned off the ready energy created by the spleen, or digestive system.

In modern terms, someone who needs a "caffeine fix," a "sugar high," or a cigarette to deal with a decision or a mental task would be especially susceptible to this energy imbalance. The digestive system cannot supply energy to the lungs, and over time *ki* stagnates in the chest. While centuries of Kampo practitioners have seen this energy imbalance as the principle cause of chest painful obstruction syndrome, Kampo also recognizes that chest pain can result from recurrent infections, excessive consumption of fats, sweets, dairy foods, or raw or cold foods, and old age. Heart pain, such as angina, is only a severe manifestation of this basic energy imbalance.

Documentation

Laboratory experimentation at the Kampo Research Laboratories of Kanebo Corporation in Japan has found that Ginseng Formula to Nourish the Nutritive *Qi* helps the body preserve cortisols. These hormones, which include adrenaline, are natural anti-inflammatory agents that reduce swelling and relieve pain[1] Other research sponsored by the Kanebo Corporation found that the formula helps correct T-cell deficiencies in animals.[2] Studies with human volunteers at the Shimane Institute, also in Japan, found that it boost natural-killer (NK) cell response to infection.[3]

Comparisons to Other Formulas

Astragalus Formula may be more effective when there is anemia and/or mild abdominal pain.

Restore the Spleen Formula may be more effective when insomnia due to shallow sleep is a major symptom.

Ten-Significant Tonic Decoction may be more effective for similar symptoms, except cough.

Goddess Powder

Japanese Name: Nyoshin-san
Chinese Name: Nu Shen San
Scientific Name: Pulvis divinatatis veni

Common Brand Names

Dang Gui & Cyperus (Qualiherb)
Fu Kang (ProBotanixx)
Nu Shen San (ProBotanixx, Qualiherb, Sun Ten)
Nyoshin-san (Honso,* Tsumura*)
Nyoshinsan Formula 035 (Kampo Institute*)
Tang-kuei & Cyperus Formula (Sun Ten)
(* Made in Japan)

Herbs Used to Make a Single Dose

Cyperus Rhizoma 3.0 g
Ligusticum Rhizome 3.0 g
Atracylodis Rhizome 3.0 g
Angelica Root 3.0 g
Scutellaria Root 3.0 g
Cinnamon Bark 2.0 g
Ginseng 2.0 g
Betel Nut 2.0 g
Coptis Rhizome 1.0 g
Licorice Root 1.0 g
Carophyllis Flower 1.0 g
Saussurea Root 1.0 g

Health Conditions Treated

Anxiety, depression, hypochondria (considered to be a physical disease by Kampo), discomforts of menopause, menstrual irregularities, PMS, and vaginal infections.

Who Should Use This Formula?

Women or men in relatively good physical condition.

Consider This Formula If You Have Any of the Health Conditions Listed Above and Experience

Feeling of uprising heat, vertigo, headache, heavy feeling of the head, palpitation, insomnia, lower back pain, and/or preoccupation with illness.

Energy Diagnosis

This formula is appropriate for an energy diagnosis of:

- Second Stage of Disease
- *Ki* neither deficient nor excessive
- *Oketsu*
- Yang excess in the liver (excessive outward energy of emotion) and heart (excessive thought)

Explanation

This formula was devised as a tonic to treat Yin deficiencies in the kidneys. A lack of "containing" energies in the kidneys results in excessive urination. The primary symptoms this formula treats, however, concern the inappropriate loss of kidney energy to other organs.

An overcharged liver results in an inability to contain the energies of emotion. There may be disturbances all along the energy channels governed by the liver, especially the breasts and the eyes. An excessively energized heart results in unrestrained emotions, words and actions that are not anchored in spirit. In both men and women, this syndrome results in a preoccupation with self and a tendency to be one's own worst enemy when under stress.

Documentation

Most of the pharmacological actions of this formula are attributable to cyperus, which is the "nut" of nutgrass. Traditional Chinese Medicine makes extensive use of cyperus in treating treat dysmenorrhea and other menstrual irregularities. Teas and tablets made from freeze-dried teas of cyperus relax the smooth muscles supporting the uterus, relieving uterine pain. While cyperus relaxes muscles surrounding the uterus, it stimulates gastric and salivary secretion, and activates the smooth muscles lining the stomach, speeding up the rate at which they propel food through the digestive tract.[1]

Laboratory tests show that cyperus improves circulation by making red blood cells more "slippery," increasing the fluidity of the blood. This action reduces the potential for swelling and varicose veins.[2]

Kudzu Formula

Japanese Name: Kakkon-to
Chinese Name: Ge Gen Tang
Scientific Name: Formula puerariae

Common Brand Names

Ge Gen Tang (Chinese Classics, Golden Flower Chinese Herbs, Honso,* Kan Traditionals, Lotus Classics, ProBotanixx, Qualiherb, Sun Ten)
Kakkon-to (Tsumura*)
Kakkonto Formula 026 (Kampo Institute*)
Kampo4Cold/Flu Pueraria Formula (Honso*)
Kudzu Releasing Formula (Kan Traditionals)
Pueraria Combination (Lotus Classics, Qualiherb, Sun Ten)
Pueraria Formula (Golden Flower Chinese Herbs)
Pueraria Plus Formula (Chinese Classics)
Shu Jin 1 (ProBotanixx)
(* Made in Japan)

Herbs Used to Make a Single Dose

Kudzu Root 4.0 g
Jujube Fruit 3.0 g
Ephedra Leaf 3.0 g
Licorice Root 2.0 g
Cinnamon Bark 2.0 g
Peony Root 2.0 g
Ginger (fresh) 2.0 g

Health Conditions Treated

Allergy, conjunctivitis, middle ear infections, hives, mastitis, and neuralgia in the upper half of the body.

Who Should Use This Formula?

Physically active individuals who experience acute upper respiratory infection, allergies, or muscle pain in the neck and shoulders.

Consider This Formula If You Have Any of the Health Conditions Listed Above and Experience

Headache, sweating alternating with chills, sudden fever, painful tension of neck muscles, upper respiratory inflammation, itch, feeling of uprising heat, red skin, conjunctivitis, and/or swollen lymph glands.

Energy Diagnosis

This formula is appropriate for an energy diagnosis of:

- First Stage of Disease
- *Ki* excess
- Yang reactions

Explanation

Kudzu Formula is a combination of herbs recommended by the venerable herbalist Zhang Zhong-jing for symptoms of the First Stage of

Disease, which he likened to "a bird that strains its neck in an attempt to fly." Colds, upper respiratory infections, allergies, and tendinitis or bursitis in the neck and shoulders bind the Yang energies as they rise to the head. The result is muscle tension and headache. The pathogenic energies of these conditions also block the flow of fluids, so there is fever, phlegm, and an absence of fever.

Documentation

Researchers in Japan recognized the metaphor of "a bird that strains . . . to fly" as descriptive of herpes infection. Most viral infections, such as colds, are eliminated by the immune system in a few days or perhaps a few weeks. The herpes virus, however, can remain in nerve tissues for many years without causing symptoms. It is activated when the body's overall resistance is weakened. The weakened immune system's only effective response to the infection is to destroy infected cells. The resulting cascade of inflammation and tissue damage can cause serious complications, and even result in death in infants and adults who are infected with both herpes and HIV.

Researchers at Toyama University in Japan studied the use of Kudzu Decoction as a herpes treatment. Their research found that the formula neither kills the virus directly nor activates the body's immune system. Instead, Kudzu Decoction blocks the tissue-damaging effects of the reactivated virus.[1] In this way, the traditional Chinese herbal formula treats one disease without creating a worse condition in its place.

Kudzu Decoction alleviates herpes outbreaks and also protects skin damaged by eczema or psoriasis from herpes infection.[2] It is also used in everyday treatment in Japan for nasal allergy or colds accompanied by stiff neck or back, diarrhea and food allergies in children, ear infections, and sinusitis.

Note: While this formula is extraordinarily non-toxic, it is important to drink at least eight glasses of water a day while taking bottled versions of the formula to avoid a small risk of dehydration.

Ledebouriella Powder That Sagely Unblocks

This formula is, as its name suggests, a combination of herbs of which ledebouriella is the chief ingredient. Ledebouriella acts "sagely" in that it restores the normal circulation of energies and fluids to the upper parts of the body without taxing the immune system.

Japanese Name: Bofu-tsusho-san
Chinese Name: Fang Feng Tong Sheng San
Scientific Name: Pulvis ledebouriellae compositae

Common Brand Names

Astra 18 Diet Fuel (Health Concerns)
Bofu-tsusho-san (Tsumura*)
Bufutsushosan Formula 034 (Kampo Institute*)
Fang Feng Tong Sheng San (Health Concerns, Honso,* Lotus Classics, Qualiherb, Sun Ten)
Kampo2Slim Slender Plus (Honso*)
Ledebouriella & Platycodon (Qualiherb)
Siler & Platycodon Formula (Lotus Classics, Sun Ten)
(* Made in Japan)

Herbs Used to Make a Single Dose

Scutellaria Root 2.0 g
Licorice Root 2.0 g
Platycodon Root 2.0 g
Gypsum 2.0 g
Wild Angelica Root 2.0 g
Rhubarb Root 1.5 g
Schizonepeta (Japanese mint) spikes 1.2 g
Gardenia Fruit 1.2 g

Peony Root 1.2 g
Ligusticum Rhizome 1.2 g
Angelica Root 1.2 g
Mint Leaf and Stems 1.2 g
Ledebouriella Root 1.2 g
Ephedra Leaf 1.2 g
Forsythia Fruit 1.2 g
Ginger (fresh) 0.3 g
Kadinum (medicinal clay) 3.0 g
Epsom Salts 0.7 g

Health Conditions Treated

"Beer belly" obesity and hypertension.

Who Should Use This Formula?

Overweight persons whose weight is concentrated over the stomach.

Consider This Formula If You Have Any of the Health Conditions Listed Above and Experience

Obesity, hypertension, racing heart, painful tension of the neck muscles, feeling of uprising heat, and/or chronic constipation.

Energy Diagnosis

This formula is appropriate for an energy diagnosis of:

- Third Stage of Disease
- Yang status causing heat in the interior layers of the body
- Localized *ki* excess

Explanation

This formula was recorded in the twelfth century as a remedy for acne, boils, and carbuncles. Over the past century, Kampo physicians have recognized that certain kinds of obesity are the result of the same kind of energy disturbances as those causing skin outbreaks. The treatment of obesity has become the primary application of this formula.

In Kampo theory, some cases of obesity begin as "overheating" in the middle of the body. As long as the overheating is the result of an overactive metabolism, the body is able to cope with excess energy by physical activity, nervous fidgeting, and sweating. Sooner or later, however, an external source of heat, usually an infection, is more than the body's natural cooling systems can handle. Heat rises to the upper parts of the body, causing any of a variety of symptoms including acne, eczema, dry mouth, flushes, or headache.

In this condition, the inability of the heart to send *ki* to the taste buds results in loss of appetite. As a result, the person constantly nibbles and snacks and picks at food, consuming more and more calories with less and less nourishment. The body is deprived of the full measure of *ki* a balanced meal provides so the muscles become weak and there is constant fatigue. On the other hand, *loss* of appetite has led to excessive consumption of food and there is weight gain.

In addition to weight gain, Ledebouriella Powder that Sagely Unblocks treats a variety of symptoms of energy congestion in the upper reaches of the body. These include a bitter taste in the mouth, focused pain in the chest, and nasal congestion. It also treats a variety of symptoms resulting from the failure to consume adequate volumes of fluid: constipation, dark urine, and elevated cholesterol.

Documentation

The herb ledebouriella has an inhibitory effect against some flu viruses as well as the bacteria that cause pseudomonas, shigella, and staph infections. Taken in teas, it relieves fever. Since approximately 450 scientific studies over the past ten years point to a viral cause of obesity in animals and people, it is plausible (but not proven) that Ledebouriella Powder that Sagely Unblocks helps stop the process of weight gain through an antiviral effect. Ledebouriella teas also lower the sensitivity of the nervous system to pain.[1]

Laboratory studies of animals suggest that obese animals have defects in the production of endogenous opioids—natural painkillers.

It is plausible, but not proven, that Ledebouriella Powder could help treat obesity by restoring normal responses to pain.

What laboratory science has confirmed is that the formula activates energy-burning brown fat cells. In experiments with laboratory animals, the formula reduces both percent body fat and total body weight without changes in the number of calories consumed.[2] Animal studies also suggest that Ledebouriella Powder keeps sugar from being deposited as fat and lowers both blood sugars and triglycerides in diabetes.[3] It speeds up the metabolism to burn fat without exercise.

Comparisons to Other Formulas

White Tiger Formula with Ginseng may be more effective for the symptoms Ledebouriella Powder that Sagely Unblocks treats when there is also thirst.

Licorice, Wheat, and Jujube Formula

Japanese Name: Kanbaku-taiso-to
Chinese Name: Gan Mai Da Zao Tang
Scientific Name: Formula zizyphi tritici glycyrrhizae

Common Brand Names

Gan Mai Da Zao Tang (Herbal Times, Kan Traditionals, Lotus Classics, Qualiherb, Sun Ten)
Kanbaku-taiso-to (Honso,* Tsumura*)
Licorice & Jujube Combination (Lotus Classics, Qualiherb, Sun Ten)
Rescue Formula (Kan Traditionals)
(* Made in Japan)

Herbs Used to Make a Single Dose

Jujube Fruit 6.0 g
Licorice Root 5.0 g
Wheat 20.0 g

Health Conditions Treated

Anxiety and nighttime fear in small children, fearfulness and fits of crying in small children, hypochondria, hysteria, insomnia, emotional instability during menopause, and emotional shock.

Who Should Use This Formula?

Children and adults who tend to be physically weak and/or inactive.

Consider This Formula If You Have Any of the Health Conditions Listed Above and Experience

Fearfulness, restlessness, muscle spasms, tendency for cramps, and/or repeated yawning. In adults: phases of depression changing with exhilaration, pessimism even though condition is improving.

Energy Diagnosis

This formula is appropriate for an energy diagnosis of:

- Second Stage of Disease
- Yang deficiency
- *Ki* deficiency

Explanation

This formula treats what Traditional Chinese Medicine calls "restless organ disorder." In this condition, anxiety, worry, or mental preoccupation injure the heart Yin, disrupt the flow of liver *ki*, and deplete the energies of the spleen. Energy accumulates in the stomach, depleting fire in the heart and reducing the amount of energy available for orderly thought processes. This generalized disruption of the internal organs by the energies of anxiety often causes recurring blood loss, which further aggravates the underlying imbalance.

The causes of this condition are emotional, and the results of this condition are also emotional. In the early stages of the syndrome, the person is anxious, disoriented, and impulsive, and suffers insomnia. During acute attacks of this syndrome, the person is upset to the point of uncontrollable crying, disorientation, or manic behavior. Kampo medicine explains this condition as a futile attempt of the Yang of the body to reunite with the Yin. Restoring balance eventually becomes impossible without intervention of acupuncture and/or herbal medicine.

Documentation

The gluten in wheat at one time was thought to have pharmacological actions similar to those of opium on the brain. Recent research has found that a protein in wheat gluten acts as part of the nervous system outside the brain to lower the threshold of pain. Laboratory animals given wheat gluten do not experience pain as quickly under conditions of stress. In the brain, the same protein seems to enhance memory and make learning faster.[1]

Comparisons to Other Formulas

Bupleurum, Dragon Bone, and Oyster Shell Formula may be more effective when there is muscular tension and emotional symptoms seem to be "bursts" of previously unexpressed emotions.

Cinnamon and Oyster Shell Formula may be more effective when there is a marked imbalance in *ki* distribution, causing fits of sweating.

Major Bupleurum Formula

In Kampo medicine, a "major" formula is given when a "minor" formula for treating the same symptom pattern has not been successful.

Japanese Name: Dai-saiko-to
Chinese Name: Da Chai Hu Tang
Scientific Name: Formula bupleuri major

Common Brand Names

Da Chai Hu Tang (Lotus Classics, Qualiherb, Sun Ten)
Dai-saiko-to (Honso,* Tsumura*)
Daisaikoto Formula 023 (Kampo Institute*)
Major Bupleurum Combination (Lotus Classics, Qualiherb, Sun Ten)
(* Made in Japan)

Herbs Used to Make a Single Dose

Bupleurum Root 6.0 g
Pinellia Tuber 4.0 g
Peony Root 3.0 g
Jujube Fruit 3.0 g
Bitter Orange (whole) 2.0 g
Ginger (fresh) 12.0 g
Rhubarb Root 1.0 g
Scutellaria Root 3.0 g

Health Conditions Treated

Acid reflux, chronic hepatitis, cirrhosis of the liver, eczema, gallstones, gallbladder pain, hemorrhoids, hives, hypertension, and tinnitus.

Who Should Use This Formula?

Strong persons with a tendency for obesity.

Consider This Formula If You Have Any of the Health Conditions Listed Above and Experience

Constipation, painful tension of neck and shoulder muscles, bloating and gas, headache with a feeling of heaviness in the head, dizziness, tinnitus, feeling of uprising heat, restlessness, nervousness, and/or tension in the abdominal muscles.

Energy Diagnosis

This formula is appropriate for an energy diagnosis of:

- Second Stage of Disease
- *Ki* congestion causing localized *ki* deficiency in the chest and weakness in the "spleen" (digestive function)

Explanation

Major Bupleurum Formula was an invention of Zhang Zhong-jing for treating conditions in which Minor Bupleurum Formula had been only partly successful. Doctor Zhang gave Minor Bupleurum Formula for the Third Stage of Disease. Sometimes patients taking Minor Bupleurum Formula for a few days then showed symptoms of the Second Stage of Disease, for which Zhang prescribed Major Bupleurum Formula.

Like other formulas containing bupleurum, Major Bupleurum Formula treats "half-exterior, half-interior" diseases. When use of Minor Bupleurum Formula enables the person to return to the Second Stage of Disease, the disease-causing energy has weakened but not entirely succumbed to the action of the herbs. Sometimes "right *ki*" prevails, and there is a feeling of heat radiating out of the body to "sweat out" the disease. Sometimes "evil *ki*" prevails, and there is a sensation of chilling cold. The symptoms of uncontrolled vomiting, despondency, and irritability will be more severe in patients who have returned to the Second Stage of Disease than in patients whose condition never progressed past the Second Stage of Disease.

The herbs in this formula are specifically helpful for disorders of the gallbladder and stomach. Vomiting treated by these herbs resulted from a reactivation of gallbladder energy overwhelming the stomach, rather than an inherent energy disorder in the stomach itself.

Documentation

Major Bupleurum Decoction has been analyzed in at least twenty-seven scientific studies. It reduces the rate at which glucose enters the bloodstream from digested food after meals and increases the efficiency of insulin.[1] It is especially useful for treatment of persons who have diabetes with long-term gastrointestinal disorders such as gastroparesis. The formula also reduces concentration of cholesterol in the bile, inhibiting the formation of gallstones.[2]

Clinical research establishes that Major Bupleurum Decoction is useful for people who have problems with both overweight and high cholesterol. A study found that a three-month course of treatment with this formula usually raises HDL ("good") cholesterol and lowers LDL ("bad") cholesterol while also preventing free radical reactions than can lead to atherosclerosis.[3] At least one laboratory study suggests Major Bupleurum Decoction is capable of reducing damage to nerve tissue after heart attack and stroke. It achieves this effect by scavenging oxygen-derived free radicals that are formed when blood circulation is restored after blood clots dissolve.[4]

Comparisons to Other Formulas

Bupleurum and Cinnamon Formula may be more effective when there is no tension in the abdominal muscles, but there is tension above the belly button.

Frigid Extremities Powder may be more effective when symptoms include cold hands and feet.

Major Construct the Middle Formula

Japanese Name: Dai-kenchu-to
Chinese Name: Da Jian Zhong Tang
Scientific Name: Formula salubritatis abdominis major

Common Brand Names

Da Jian Zhong Tang (Lotus Classics, Qualiherb, Sun Ten)
Dai-kenchu-to (Honso,* Tsumura*)
Major Zanthoxylum Combination (Lotus Classics, Qualiherb, Sun Ten)
(* Made in Japan)

Herbs Used to Make a Single Dose

Ginseng 3.0 g
Zanthoxylum (Szechuan Pepper) 2.0 g
Ginger (dried) 5.0 g

Chinese-made formulations of this product usually incorporate an amount of malt sugar at least equal to the weight of the herbs. Chinese medical texts warn that taking this formula with cane sugar rather than malt sugar will ruin its effects. Japanese-made formulations of this product usually omit sugar entirely.

Health Conditions Treated

Bloating, chronic enteritis, flatulence, gallstones, gallbladder pain, irritable bowel syndrome, kidney stones, and pain from peritoneal adhesions.

Who Should Use This Formula?

Physically weak persons who experience coldness in the abdomen or hands and feet.

Consider This Formula If You Have Any of the Health Conditions Listed Above and Experience

Bloating, noticeable pain in the abdomen without tension of the abdominal muscles, or spasms in the lower stomach.

Energy Diagnosis

This formula is appropriate for an energy diagnosis of:

- Fourth Stage of Disease
- *Ki* deficiency
- Yin excess, especially in the intestine

Explanation

This formula uses an exceptionally "hot" herb, Szechuan pepper, to treat exceptionally "cold" diseases. In the symptom pattern for which this combination of herbs was designed, repeated infection, a diet containing too many sugary or greasy foods, or excessive exposure to cold temperatures (either winter cold or air conditioning) has depleted Yang energies throughout the body. The body reacts to a deficiency of Yang with an excess of Yin, sending Yin energies upward from the digestive tract to organs that are attuned to Yang. The result of confused energies is pain. The pain in the abdomen and epigastric regions may be so intense that the person cannot bear to be touched. There may be rumbling fluids in the stomach followed by vomiting so severe it becomes impossible for the patient to eat.

Zhang Zhong-jing thought it was very important to correct this syndrome with malt sugar, made from the "five grains of nourishment." Malt sugar, but not cane sugar, was thought to restore the nutrients that the body had lost by vomiting and needed immediately. Kampo medicines do not contain malt sugar, but Japanese physicians sometimes recommend patients with this symptom pattern take additional fruit juices when vomiting stops.

Documentation

Clinical research in Japan has found that Major Construct the Middle Formula increases the digestive tract's supply of the protein 5-HTP.[1] This protein is a source of the amino acid trytophan in a form that is readily absorbed by nerves both in the digestive tract and in the brain. The nervous system turns trytophan into the mood regulator serotonin. The digestive tract uses serotonin to signal the brain when something is wrong, such as bloating or muscle spasms. The formula also stimulates the release of other neurogregulators that make sure digested food passes from the stomach into the intestine quickly, with a minimal production of acid.

Japanese doctors have explored the use of this formula in treating pelvic adhesions occurring after gynecological surgery. These internal scars cause constipation that cannot be treated with fiber or laxatives. Major Construct the Middle Formula acts on muscles that are not affected by laxatives so that the bowels can move. Laboratory testing suggests that the formula does not affect the uterus, so that it is safe for use by pregnant women.[2]

Minor Bluegreen Dragon Decoction

In Chinese folk religion, Seiryu, the bluegreen dragon, was the wood spirit from the east. He was present in the billowing ocean waves and responsible for generating clouds as well as causing them to release rain. A major bluegreen dragon caused rain, while a minor bluegreen dragon stirred the waves, in this case, waves of relief.

Japanese Name: Sho-seiryu-to
Chinese Name: Xiao Qing Long Tang
Scientific Name: Formula divinitatis caerulea minor

Common Brand Names

Minor Blue Dragon Formula (Chinese Classics)
Minor Blue Dragon (Health Concerns, Qualiherb)
Minor Blue Dragon Combination (Lotus Classics)
Sho-seiryu-to (Honso,* Tsumura*)
(* Made in Japan)

Herbs Used to Make a Single Dose

Pinellia Tuber 6.0 g
Licorice Root 3.0 g
Cinnamon Bark 30
Schisandra Fruit 3.0 g
Asiasarum Root 3.0 g
Peony Root 3.0 g
Ephedra Leaf 3.0 g
Ginger (dried) 3.0 g

Health Conditions Treated

Asthma, bronchitis, colds, and flu.

Who Should Use This Formula?

Physically strong persons suffering respiratory distress.

Consider This Formula If You Have Any of the Health Conditions Listed Above and Experience

Cough, shortness of breath, wheezing, foamy phlegm, runny nose, fever, and/or rumbling sounds in the digestive tract.

Energy Diagnosis

This formula is appropriate for an energy diagnosis of:

- First Stage of Disease
- Yang excess

- *Ki* deficiency
- Cold localized in the "middle" of the body

Chronic stasis of fluids also contributes to this syndrome, but is not always evident at the same time as respiratory symptoms.

Explanation

Minor Bluegreen Dragon Formula is an herb combination recorded in a passage in Zhang Zhong-jing's *Treatise on Infectious Cold* that is particularly difficult to understand. Doctor Zhang gave no fewer than seven variations of this formula for subtle variations in symptoms. He referred to herbs that are used nowhere else in Kampo medicine. Modern-day translators speculate that the parchments of the ancient text recording this formula were damaged and later copyists were left to guess the master's intentions.

Whatever the "true" recipe for this formula might be, today it is used to treat upper respiratory infections in people who have a tendency for disturbed fluid metabolism. The people whose bronchitis, colds, and flu this formula treats especially well are people who tend to have bloating, water retention, or urinary difficulties. The Kampo theory of how these herbs work is based on the observation that people who have congested fluids tend to have weak lungs. When they contract a respiratory infection, their lungs cannot "cough out" the invading microorganism, so the bacterium or virus takes hold. As the infection worsens, congested fluids "congeal" into white stringy sputum that is difficult to cough up, creating a stifling sensation in the chest. In severe cases, it is difficult to breathe while lying down.

Documentation

One of the problems with flu shots is that the makers of the vaccine have to guess which strain of influenza will be most common the next winter. Laboratory tests with animals have found that Minor Bluegreen Dragon formula induces changes in the immune system that create cross-protection against not just one but multiple strains of both inluenza A virus and influenza B virus.[1] A double-blind clinical study involving 220 participants in Japan also confirmed that Minor Bluegreen Dragon Formula can relieve the symptoms of seasonal allergies, including runny nose and sinus congestion. (The formula was slightly more effective for relieving sinus congestion than for relieving runny nose).[2] Although the formula act an antihistamine, it does not cause drowsiness or irregular pulse.[3]

Minor Bupleurum Formula

A "minor" formula uses the smallest effective number of herbs in the first attempt to treat a disease.

Japanese Name: Sho-saiko-to
Chinese Name: Xiao Chai Hu Tang
Scientific Name: Formula bupeluri minor

Common Brand Names

Sho-saiko-to (Honso,* Tsumura*)
Minor Bupleurum Formula (Chinese Classics, Golden Flower Chinese Herbs)
Minor Bupleurum Formulation (Kan Traditionals)
Minor Bupleurum Combination (Lotus Classics, Qualiherb, Sun Ten)
Liver Kampo (Honso*)
Xiao Chai Hu Tang (Chinese Classics, Golden Flower Chinese Herbs, Herbal Times, Honso,* Kan Traditionals, Lotus Classics, Qualiherb, Sun Ten)
(* Made in Japan)

Herbs Used to Make a Single Dose

Bupleurum Root 7.0 g
Pinellia Tuber 5.0 g
Ginseng 3.0 g
Jujube Fruit 3.0 g
Licorice Root 2.0 g
Ginger (dried) 1.0 g
Scutellaria Root 3.0 g

Health Conditions Treated

Bronchitis, chronic hepatitis, cirrhosis of the liver, and liver cancer.

Who Should Use This Formula?

Individuals who are physically able to continue their daily routines despite chronic illness.

Consider This Formula If You Have Any of the Health Conditions Listed Above and Experience

Loss of appetite, nausea, and/or periods of exhaustion due to chronic disease.

Energy Diagnosis

This formula is appropriate for an energy diagnosis of:

- Second Stage of Disease
- Yang Deficiency
- *Ki* neither deficient nor excessive

Explanation

Minor Bupleurum Formula treats diseases that are "half in" and "half out" of the body. These are disease conditions that may be quiescent for many years before exploding into a panoply of serious and even life-threatening symptoms. Viral hepatitis is a disease in this category. Historically, Kampo physicians recognized the presence of a "half-in, half-out" condition by digestive symptoms. Long-term infections of this class that are about to progress to a more serious state produce three classes of symptoms:

- Alternating chills and fever with a sensation of fullness in the chest
- Bitter or sour taste in the mouth, sore throat, or dizziness
- Heartburn, nausea, vomiting, and reduced appetite

Documentation

Nearly 200 scientific studies have looked into various aspects of the efficacy of Minor Bupleurum Decoction, also widely known by its Japanese name, sho-saiko-to. This herbal formula has become the most widely used natural treatment for hepatitis B. In the late 1980s clinical trials in Japan established that taking the formula for twelve weeks lowered concentrations of the hepatitis B virus in the bloodstream and reduced the rates of liver damage.[1] Laboratory tests have found that taking both Minor Bupleurum Decoction and vaccine results in a 100 percent rate of remission from hepatitis B infection (compared to nine to ten percent for either the herbal formula or the vaccine alone).[2] In hepatitis C, Minor Bupleurum Decoction slows the formation of fibrous tissue in the liver and can greatly slow the progression of the disease.[3]

The most exciting application of Minor Bupleurum Decoction, however, is its potential in treating liver cancer. The formula seems to stop the growth of tumors rather than to kill tumor cells (which would require the immune system to isolate the dead cancer cells with inflammation and "fill in" the space occupied by the tumor with scar tissue). As this book is being written, eighty liver cancer patients at the Memorial Sloan-Kettering Cancer Center in New York are being treated with 7.5 grams of the herbal formula, a day, their progress with the treatment to evaluated in August 2002 and May 2003.

Warnings: Do not take this formula during fever. In addition, Japanese physicians have reported over 100 cases of interstitial pneumonia (pneumonia causing congestion lower in the lungs than in bronchitis) among hepatitis C patients being treated with *both* Minor Bupleurum

Formula and interferon. In these cases, pneumonia is an unusual complication of immune over-stimulation. Discontinue this formula immediately if you experience chest pain or difficulty breathing.

Polyporus Formula

Japanese Name: Chorei-to
Chinese Name: Zhu Ling Tang
Scientific Name: Formula polypori

Common Brand Names

Chorei-to (Tsumura*)
Polyporus Combination (Lotus Classics, Sun Ten)
Zhu Ling Tang (Lotus Classics, Sun Ten)
(* Made in Japan)

Herbs Used to Make a Single Dose

Polyporus 3.0 g
Poria 3.0 g
Alisma Rhizome 3.0 g
Donkey Hide Gelatin 3.0 g
Kadinum (medicinal clay) 3.0 g
Some Japanese-made preparations use agar instead of donkey-hide gelatin in order to meet kosher requirements.

Health Conditions Treated

Difficult urination, inflammation of the urinary tract, kidney stones, and gonorrhea.

Who Should Use This Formula?

Persons whose urinary problems have lasted a month or longer.

Consider This Formula If You Have Any of the Health Conditions Listed Above and Experience

A feeling of incomplete urination, inflammation of the urinary tract, thirst, and/or diarrhea.

Energy Diagnosis

This formula is appropriate for an energy diagnosis of:

- Third or Fourth Stage of Disease
- Localized heat in the urinary tract resulting from pathogenic cold (infection) transforming itself into heat
- Stasis of fluids
- Overall *ki* neither deficient nor excessive

Explanation

This formula treats a condition in which an infection has entered the "middle" layers of the body, specifically the urinary tract, and induced the body to respond with heat. Heat battles with water in the urinary tract and causes "clumps," blocking the normal flow of urine. If the infection has induced the Fourth Stage of Disease, it also interferes with the flow of *ki* to the legs, causing swollen feet and aggravating varicose veins and cellulite.

Heat causes fever, and fever gives rise to thirst. If a person with this syndrome attempts to assuage fever by drinking fluids, the kidneys cannot eliminate them as urine. Fluids must be expelled with the stool, resulting in diarrhea. Over time, the disturbance of fluid metabolism disturbs the lungs, and there will be coughing, due not to a respiratory infection but symptomatic of urinary tract infection.

Documentation

Japanese medicine has considerable experience in using Polyporus Formula to treat urinary tract infections. Tsumura & Company confirms that approximately two-thirds of female patients who have a combination of symptoms modern Japanese doctors call "urethral syndrome"—painful urination and/or a sense of incomplete urination—improve when taking this formula. About six percent of patients experience some degree of stomach upset when first taking the formula, but this side effect is not so great that they choose to discontinue the herbs.

Polyporus Formula also accelerates the passage of kidney stones. It is important to note that the effect of the herbs on kidney stones is highly dependent on dosage. Modern Chinese formulas employ two to three times the amount of herbs specified in by Zhang Zhong-jing. Clinical tests of Polyporus Decoction show that at "Japanese" dosages, the formula relieves kidney stones without forcing the body to excrete vitamin C, unlike most medications for kidney stones. "Chinese" higher doses of the formula, however, have no effect on kidney stones.[1] Whether or not the passage of kidney stones is desirable is a matter for the patient's and the physician's judgment.

Comparisons to Other Formulas

Five-Ingredient Powder for Painful Urinary Dysfunction may be more effective if there is inflammation of the urinary tract with severe pain.

Lotus Seed Formula to Clear the Kidneys may be more effective if there is a burning sensation during urination.

Warning: This formula is not appropriate during *acute* pain of kidney stones, but instead should be used long-term as a preventive measure.

Relax the Channels and Invigorate the Blood Formula

Japanese Name: Sokei-kakketsu-to

Chinese Name: Shu Jing Huo Xue Tang

Scientific Name: Formula augmentationis orbis et cruorem dissolvans

Common Brand Names

Clematis & Stephania Combination (Lotus Classics)
Clematis & Stephania Formula (Chinese Classics)
Mobility 2 (Health Concerns)
Shu Jin Huo Xue Tang (Chinese Classics, Golden Flower Chinese Herbs, Health Concerns, Lotus Classics)
Sokei-kakketsu-to (Honso,* Tsumura*)
Sokeikakketsuto Formula 031 (Kampo Institute*)
(* Made in Japan)

Herbs Used to Make a Single Dose

Peony Root 3.5 g
Rehmannia Root 2.0 g
Ligusticum Rhizome 2.0 g
White Atractylodis Rhizome 2.0 g
Angelica Root 2.0 g
Peach Seed 2.0 g
Poria 2.0 g
Evodia Fruit 1.5 g
Chen-Pi Peel 1.5 g
Sinomenium Caulus and Rhizome 21.5 g
Ledebouriella Root 1.5 g
Gentian Root 1.5 g
Licorice Root 1.0 g
Wild Angelica Root 1.0 g

Ginger (fresh) 0.5 g
Clematis Root 1.5 g
Notopterygium Rhizome 1.5 g

Health Conditions Treated

Back pain (especially in the coccyx, or tail bone).

Who Should Use This Formula?

Relatively strong persons who experience lower back pain and who have freckles, age spots, or other areas of dark pigmentation on the skin.

Consider This Formula If You Have Any of the Health Conditions Listed Above and Experience

Back pain, cold limbs, swollen scrotum in men, and/or areas of dark pigmentation on the skin.

Energy Diagnosis

This formula is appropriate for an energy diagnosis of:

- Second Stage of Disease
- Yang deficiency
- *Ki* deficiency
- Oketsu

Explanation

This formula is a variation on an herbal tea devised by a nineteenth-century Chinese physician, Wang Qing-Ren. In his book, *Correction of Errors Among Physicians*, Wang proposed a formula he called Tonify the Yang to Restore Five-Tenths Decoction. Wang believed that a stroke affecting one side of the body took away five-tenths of the body's yang energies. However, Wang recalled that some conditions seemed to be the opposite of stroke, that is, the body's Yang was excessive by five-tenths rather than deficient by five-tenths. For these conditions, which included back pain, age spots, and scrotal hernia, he recommended a formula by the sixteenth century physician Gong Ting-Xian recorded in *Recovery from Myriad Diseases*, called Relax the Channels and Invigorate the Blood Formula.

Relaxing the channels and invigorating the blood refers to the restoration of channels clogged with Yang energy the immune system has mustered to fight "wind-dampness." Pathogenic wind, cold and dampness fight against one another in the blood vessels and attack the heart, obstructing its vessels and hindering the smooth circulation of the blood, thus resulting in palpitations. However, as wind-dampness disease progresses, the body produces Yang that collides with the pathogenic energy and causes painful obstruction in the lower back and legs, or pigmentation of the skin.

Traditional Chinese Medicine physician Bob Flaws notes that in this syndrome it is especially important to avoid misuse of ginseng. This Yang tonic herb can generate energies that induce more "dampness" and aggravate lower back pain.

Documentation

While Relax the Channels and Invigorate the *Qi* Formula has been used with success in clinical practice throughout East Asia for nearly 150 years, only the slightest scientific evidence exists of its mechanism of action. Japanese scientists seeking treatments for radiation exposure found that this formula acts as a free-radical scavenger and prevents tissue damage from radiation burns.[1] It is possible, but not proven, that the formula acts in a similar way to stop hormonal reactions that cause pain and inflammation in throughout the body.

Comparisons to Other Formulas

Five-Accumulation Powder may be more effective when there are chills, headache, diarrhea, and/or abdominal pain.

Six-Ingredient Pill with Rehmannia

Practitioners of Traditional Chinese Medicine frequently refer to this formula as Rehmannia-Six Combination.

Japanese Name: Rokumi-jio-gan
Chinese Name: Liu Wei Di Huang Wan
Scientific Name: Formula medicamentorum sextorum rehmanniae

Common Brand Names

Liu We Di Haung Wan (Asian Patents, Chinese Classics, Golden Flower Chinese Herbs, Health Concerns, Herbal Times, Jade Dragon, Kan Herbals, KPC Herbs, Lotus Classics, Qualiherb, Sun Ten)
Nine-Flavor Tea (Health Concerns)
Nourish Essence Formula (Golden Flower Chinese Herbs)
Quiet Contemplative (Kan Herbals)
Rehmannia 6 (Qualiherb)
Rehmannia Six Formula (KPC Herbs, Lotus Classics, Sun Ten)
Six-Flavor Tea (Asian Patents, Herbal Times)
Six-flavor Tea Formula (Jade Dragon)

Herbs Used to Make a Single Dose

Rehmannia Root 5.0 g
Cornelian Cherry Fruit 3.0 g
Dioscorea Root 3.0 g
Alisma Rhizome 3.0 g
Poria 3.0 g
Moutan Root 3.0 g

Health Conditions Treated

Asthma in children, erectile dysfunction, and excessive urination. Used in modern Traditional Chinese Medicine to treat symptoms of diabetes, failure to thrive, hyperthyroidism, and uterine bleeding.

Who Should Use This Formula?

Physically weak persons with obvious symptoms of disease.

Consider This Formula If You Have Any of the Health Conditions Listed Above and Experience

Easy fatigue, nocturnal urination, feeling of incomplete urination, lower back pain, reduced abdominal tension in the lower abdomen, sensitivity to cold but hot or sweaty hands and feet, and/or tendency for swelling.

Energy Diagnosis

This formula is appropriate for an energy diagnosis of:

- Fourth Stage of Disease
- Stasis of fluids

Explanation

Six-Ingredient Pill with Rehmannia is Kampo's most important formula for harmonizing the energies of the kidneys, heart, and liver. Modern commentators on Kampo see the common energy pattern of conditions as diverse as asthma in children and erectile dysfunction in men as an energy trace left by guilt, fear, or shock.

A feeling of guilt harbored for many years is especially damaging to the kidneys, which lose Yin, their ability to contain. In children there may be a disturbance of fluid metabolism that eventually overwhelms the lungs' ability to send energy upward. The lungs are eventually only capable of wheezing and accumulate stringy phlegm. In mature men, the depletion of Yin results in a state in which the kidneys store insufficient energy to maintain sexual intercourse. When the kidneys eventually cannot contain enough fluid to regulate the "fire" of the heart, a number of "hot" or "burning" symptoms arise. They express themselves in diseases as various as diabetic retinopathy, hyperthyroidism, optic neuritis, retinitis pigmentosa, and wasting from uncontrolled diabetes.

The most frequent application of this formula in modern Chinese medicine, however, lies in its use in treating the Five Developmental Delays—failures to thrive and pass milestones of normal growth in children. Chinese medicine has used this formula to treat delays in childhood development since it was recorded by the physician *Qian* Yi in *Craft of Medicinal Treatment for Childhood Diseases* in 1119. The Five Developmental Delays include retardation of:

- Cutting teeth.
- Developing speech.
- Growing hair on the head.
- Standing up.
- Walking.

Documentation

Dr. Margaret Naeser, an expert in Kampo patent medicines, has published case studies documenting success in using Six-Ingredient Pill with Rehmannia to treat the Five Delays in children with cerebral palsy or ADD.[1] The formula's salutary effect on intellectual development is probably due to the inclusion of poria. Some of the complex sugars in the mushroom reduce the immune system's production of cytokines,[2] inflammatory chemicals that cause anxiety, memory loss, and seizures.

Comparisons to Other Formulas

Eight-Ingredient Pill with Rehmannia may be more effective when symptoms include cold hands and feet.

Warning: This formula stimulates the production of B cells—cells of the immune system that attack the body's own tissues in rheumatoid arthritis and related conditions. For this reason, persons with rheumatoid arthritis, lupus, or Sjögren's syndrome, and especially persons with myasthenia gravis, should avoid the formula.

Stephania and Astragalus Formula

Japanese Name: Boi-ogi-to
Chinese Name: Fang Ji Huang Qi Tang
Scientific Name: Formula astragali et sinomenii

Common Brand Names

Boiogito Formula 032 (Kampo Institute*)
Fang Ji Huang Qi Tang (Kan Herbals, Lotus Classics)
Stephania & Astragalus Combination (Kan Herbals, Lotus Classics)
(* Made in Japan)

Herbs Used to Make a Single Dose

Astragalus Root 5.0 g
Sinomenium Caulus and Rhizome 5.0 g
Jujube Fruit 3.0 g
Licorice Root 1.5 g
Ginger (fresh) 1.0 g
White Atractylodis Rhizome 5.0 g

Health Conditions Treated

Anemia, arthritis, boils, excessive sweating, fatigue, and swelling of the scrotum.

Consider This Formula If You Have Any of the Health Conditions Listed Above and Experience

Pale complexion, weak muscles, swelling, sweating easily, pain and swelling of the joints, especially the knees, and/or scanty urination. Japanese physicians most commonly prescribe this formula to persons over 50 years old who do not get physical exercise and who tend to catch colds.

Energy Diagnosis

This formula is appropriate for an energy diagnosis of:

- Fourth Stage of Disease
- Yin excess
- *Ki* deficiency
- Stasis of fluids

Explanation

The pathogenic influence this formula battles is known in Chinese medicine as *feng shui*. This condition is a teaming up of the pathogenic influences of wind and water. Unlike the combination of wind and fire, the combination of wind and water in *feng shui* usually does not result in anything Western medicine would recognize as an infection. Instead, the lungs are simply unable to process damp air and take in water as well as air. If the body could generate enough protective *ki*, this would not be a problem, but generally there has been a slow wearing down of the body's immune defenses to make this impossible. People who are susceptible to *feng shui* attack usually have had allergies, tonsillitis, or recurrent respiratory infections in their younger years, and their weak respiratory system has caused them to refrain from vigorous physical activity for a period of years.

Since the pathogenic energy of wind is associated with an inability to choose or to distinguish between what is important and what is not, people who have weak lung function as children tend, in Japanese thought, to grow into nervous adults. They tend to worry too much about details, and to crave food without really being hungry and without ever feeling really satisfied. They usually prefer sweet foods and food high in liquid content. They tend to belch and release gas, and complain of pain in the shoulders and knees.

After decades of duress, the body loses its inner sense of direction with regard to fluids. In particular, the bladder loses its sense of direction with regard to fluids. A "ring of water" composed of soft, flabby, almost liquid tissue forms over the abdomen. Eventually the heaviness of water can manifest itself in other ways, such as rheumatic heart disease, ascites from liver failure, and acute and chronic nephritis.

In this final stage of *feng shui*, the entire body is in a state of Yin with systemic *ki* deficiency. Protective Yang is reduced in the exterior layers of the body, offering no protection against invasive skin infections, excessive sweating, scrotal edema, thirst, and arthritis.

Documentation

There is only one published study of Stephania and Astragalus Formula used as a whole. A Japanese study in the 1980s found that it could prevent the formation of free radicals caused by exposure to radiation in laboratory animals.[1]

The component herb astragalus, on the other hand, has been studied more extensively. In traditional Kampo medicine, the function of astragalus is to strengthen the protective *ki*. Astragalus is an effective antiviral agent,[2] and stimulates the production of natural killer (NK) cells in patients with lupus.[3] Astragalus stimulates macrophages, immune cells which surround and digest infectious microorganisms, even when it is taken in low doses.[4] These properties of astragalus partially explain the effectiveness of the formula in treating skin infections and fatigue.

Comparisons to Other Formulas

Cinnamon, Aconite, and Atractylodis Formula may be more effective when there are also muscle twitches, migraine, or convulsions.

Gypsum and Atractylodis Formula may be more effective when skin and joints are major localizations of disease.

Ledebouriella Powder that Sagely Unblocks may be more effective when there is abdominal swelling.

Ten-Herb Antidote

Japanese Name: *Jumi-haidoku-to*
Chinese Name: Shi Wei Bai Du Tang
Scientific Name: Formula decem-antidotum

Common Brand Names
Jumihaidokuto Formula 036 (Kampo Institute*)
Jumi-haidoku-to (Tsumura*)
(* Made in Japan)

Herbs Used to Make a Single Dose
Bupleurum Root 3.0 g
Platycodon Root 3.0 g
Ligusticum Rhizome 3.0 g
Poria 3.0 g
Ledebouriella Root 1.5 g
Licorice Root 1.0 g
Schizonepeta (Japanese mint) spikes 1.0 g
Ginger (dried) 1.0 g
Aralia Root and Rhizome 1.0 g
Oak Bark 3.0 g

Some versions of this formula substitute rose petals for oak bark as an astringent agent.

Health Conditions Treated
Dermatitis, eczema, and tinea (athlete's foot, inflammation around whiskers).

Who Should Use This Formula?
Physically vigorous individuals who have skin problems.

Consider This Formula If You Have Any of the Health Conditions Listed Above and Experience

Pale skin despite exposure to the sun.

Energy Diagnosis

This formula is appropriate for an energy diagnosis of:

- Second Stage of Disease
- Yang Deficiency
- *Ki* neither deficient nor excessive

Explanation

This formula treats "wind" diseases that have stagnated in the skin or sensory orifices of the body and become toxic, producing acne, boils, breast distention, carbuncles, conjunctivitis, dermatitis, eczema, swollen lymph glands, or middle-ear infections. Its astringent tannins keep infection from "oozing out" of the skin and force it to meet the immune system, which vanquishes it.

Documentation

A number of studies of the herbs from which this formula is made suggest it is an especially versatile treatment for skin inflammation. The variable ingredient in the formula is oak bark, sometimes replaced with rose petals. This herb provides tannins which tighten the skin and prevent "oozing" and inflammation. The other herbs in the formula provide a wide range of antibacterial and antiviral chemicals which stop the onslaught of infection and allow the body's immune processes to slowly overcome the disease.

Laboratory testing finds that Ten-Herb Antidote stops the inflammation that causes acne without drying out the skin, and without even killing the bacteria that cause acne. Most cleansers remove sebum, an oil secreted by the skin. Sebum keeps the skin soft and supple. It minimizes wrinkling. It enables the skin to act as a raincoat, protecting the body from water absorption through the skin. Sebum also prevents the evaporation of essential fluids from the skin. Because fat is a poor conductor of heat, sebum lessons the amount of heat loss from the body's surface in cold weather.

The acne bacterium *Propionibacterium acnes*, the same bacterium that makes the holes in Swiss cheese, feeds on excess sebum. It releases butyric and propionic acids as it digests the sebum. These acids do not eat tiny holes in the skin as long as they are free to flow to the surface, where ordinary washing with soap and water carry them away. Acne only occurs when the opening of the follicle is blocked and the acids are trapped, so they inflame the skin.

Almost every treatment for acne requires opening pores. Ten-Herb Antidote, however, works whether or not pores open. The herbal formula reduces the bacterium's production of the acids so that it can continue to cleanse the skin of excess sebum, but without causing inflammation to the skin that can lead to wrinkling later in life.[1] With Ten-Herb Antidote, even clogged pores do not result in pimples. This gives clogged pores a chance to recover on their own without disturbing any of the natural balances in the skin.

Ten-Significant Tonic Decoction

This formula is known in the popular literature as a "decoction," referring to the fact it was originally prepared by pouring boiling water over herbs. "Ten-Significant" is a literal translation of the first three characters of its name; Chinese herb books often refer to this formula as "All-Inclusive Great Tonifying Decoction," or by its name in Mandarin, Shih Qua Da Bu Tang.

Japanese Name: Juzen-taiho-to
Chinese Name: Shih Qua Da Bu Tang
Scientific Name: Formula decem-supplementorum major

Common Brand Names:

Energy Kampo (Honso*)
Ginseng & Dong Quai Ten Formula (Chinese Classics)
Ginseng & Tangkuei Ten Combination (Lotus Classics)
Ginseng & Tang-kuei Ten Combination (Sun Ten)
Juzen-taiho-to (Tsumura*)
Shih Qu Da Bu Tang (Chinese Classics, Honso,* Kan Traditionals, Lotus Classics, Qualiherb, Sun Ten)
Ten Treasures (Kan Traditionals)
(* Made in Japan)

Herbs Used to Make a Single Dose

Astragalus Root 3.0 g
Cinnamon Twig 3.0 g
Rehmannia Root 3.0 g
Peony Root 3.0 g
Ligusticum Rhizome 3.0 g
Angelica Root 3.0 g
Ginseng 3.0 g
Poria 3.0 g
Licorice Root 1.5 g
White Atractylodis Rhizome 3.0 g

Health Conditions Treated

Recuperation after surgery or chronic diseases, recuperation from extreme athletic exertion, fatigue during calorie-restricted dieting, and vitiligo.

Who Should Use This Formula?

Chemotherapy patients (with foreknowledge and approval of physician), athletes in training, and dieters.

Consider This Formula If You Have Any of the Health Conditions Listed Above and Experience

Fatigue, profuse sweating, anemia, dry skin, nightsweats, and/or dry mouth.

Energy Diagnosis

This formula is appropriate for an energy diagnosis of:

- Fourth Stage of Disease
- Marked *Ki* deficiency
- Yin Excess

Explanation

Modern Kampo medicine uses this formula to treat any disease which results in a simultaneous deficiency of blood and *ki*. The ancient herbalists who first designed this formula in the twelfth century believed that the kind of blood deficiency these herbs caused interfered with circulation to the brain. When blood flow to the brain is inadequate, headache ensues. Thinking is impaired, and the "sea of marrow" of which the brain is a part is inadequate for the health of the bones.

Documentation

Ten-Significant Tonic Decoction was one of 116 Kampo formulas screened at the University of Kansas in the early 1990s as a potential treatment for patients receiving conventional cancer therapies. There was never any intention of replacing chemotherapy or radiation therapy with Kampo. The objective of this screening was to find ways to increase survival rates and reduce patient discomforts during cancer treatment. The University of Kansas studies found that the formula was extremely nontoxic (it would be necessary to consume 1 1/2 kg, or more than three pounds, of capsules to begin to have a toxic effect). They also presented clinical data that showed that Ten-Significant Tonic Decoction:

- Stimulates the production of red blood cells during cancer chemotherapy with cisplatin, cyclophosphamide, fluorouracil, and mitomycin
- Stimulates the production of white blood cells during cancer chemotherapy with cisplatin, cyclophosphamide, fluorouracil, and mitomycin
- Reduces incidents of nausea, vomiting, general immunosuppression, and kidney damage during radiation therapy and treatment with many anti-cancer drugs[1]

Since 1992 there have been no fewer than twenty-five laboratory studies to "fine-tune" the general findings of the University of Kanasas study. Scientists at the School of Pharmaceutical Sciences at the University of Shizuoka in Japan confirmed that Ten-Significant Tonic Decoction increased red and white blood cell counts, food intake and body weight in mice treated with carboplatin and cisplatin.[2] These findings were replicated at the Kitasato Institute in Tokyo the same year. Later studies in Japan suggested that the formula prevents the metastasis of colon cancer to the liver,[3] allows the use of a smaller dose of interferon in treating kidney cancer,[4] prevents estrogen from activating endometrial cancers,[5] and activates the immune system to suppress the growth of melanoma tumors.[6] Other lines of research suggest that Ten-Significant Tonic Decoction may be as effective as estrogen in preventing osteoporosis after menopause,[7] and may counteract yeast infection.[8]

Comparisons to Other Formulas

Astragalus Formula may be taken with this formula to relieve abdominal pain.

Ginseng Formula to Nourish the Nutritive *Qi* may be taken with this formula to relieve cough and weakness of the heart.

Tonify the Middle and Augment the *Qi* Formula may be taken with this formula to relieve fever.

Tonify the Middle and Augment the Qi Formula

In Kampo medicine, a tonic relieves pathogenic cold. The "middle" refers to the digestive process in general and the stomach in particular.

Japanese Name: Hochu-ekki-to
Chinese Name: Bu Zhong Yi Qi Tang
Scientific Name: Pulvis repletionis et auxilium vis vitalis

Common Brand Names

Added Flavors Supplement the Center & Boost Qi (Blue Poppy Herbs)
Arouse Vigor (Kan Herbals)
Breaking Clouds (Three Treasures)
Bu Zhong Yi Qi Tang (Asian Patents, Blue Poppy Herbs, Chinese Classics, Golden Flower Chinese Herbs, Health Concerns, Kan Herbals, Lotus Classics, ProBotanixx, Qualiherb, Sun Ten, Three Treasures)
Central Chi Tea (Asian Patents)
Ginseng & Astragalus (Qualiherb)
Ginseng & Astragalus Combination (Sun Ten)
Ginseng & Astragalus Formula (Golden Flower Chinese Herbs)
Hochuekkito Formula 017 (Kampo Institute*)
Raise Qi (Health Concerns)
Tonify Qi & Ease the Muscles (Three Treasures)
Yi Qi (Probotanixx)
(*Made in Japan)

Herbs Used to Make a Single Dose

Astragalus Root 4.0 g
White Atractylodis Rhizome 4.0 g

Ginseng 4.0 g
Angelica Root 3.0 g
Bupleurum Root 2.0 g
Jujube Fruit 2.0 g
Chen-Pi Peel 2.0 g
Licorice Root 1.5 g
Black Cohosh Root 1.0 g
Ginger (fresh) 0.5 g

Health Conditions Treated

Chronic bronchitis, chronic hepatitis, male infertility, and prolapse of the uterus, rectum, or stomach.

Who Should Use This Formula?

Relatively weak patients with deficiency due to chronic diseases.

Consider This Formula If You Have Any of the Health Conditions Listed Above and Experience

Loss of appetite, chronic cough, mild fevers, nightsweats, palpitation, weak voice or slurred speech, and/or visual disturbances.

Energy Diagnosis

This formula is appropriate for an energy diagnosis of:

- Second Stage of Disease
- *Ki* deficiency
- Yang deficiency (Protective Yang in the exterior body, atrophy of muscles due to systemic *ki* deficiency)

Explanation

This formula treats *ki* deficiency in the "earth" organs, the spleen (digestive function) and stomach. When the person has become "ungrounded" from healthy habits regarding diet, exercise, or thought, the spleen and stomach lose their capacity to generate Yang energies. Since these organs supply energy to the muscles and the flesh, deficiency in them makes the arms and legs flabby and weak. The deficiency of Yang keeps energy from flowing to the superficial regions of the body, so there is a constant feeling of cold and fatigue.

Documentation

In the 1980s, Japanese physicians made the conceptual leap from using this formula to treat Yang-depleted limbs to using it to treat Yang-depletion causing male infertility. In a clinical study in Japan, twenty percent of participating couples achieved conception within twelve weeks, and fifty-one percent of the men taking the formula had increased sperm counts.[1] Laboratory studies with animals indicate that the formula works by stimulating the production of proteins that enable sperm to reach functional maturity. The formula is particularly effective in alleviating male reproductive problems caused by chemotherapy with doxorubin (Adriamycin).[2]

Tonify the Middle and Augment the *Qi* Formula is also used to activate the immune system to attack certain kinds of cancer. It stimulates the immune system to produce NK (natural killer) cells,[3] and it helps bone marrow recover after cancer treatment with either cyclophosphamide (Cytoxan) or radiation.[4]

True Warrior Decoction

The Japanese characters for this formula are read "true warrior" but sound the same as the words for "new warrior." In Chinese and Japanese folklore, the "true warrior" is the spirit of the north who manages both fire and water. The herbs in this formula are meant to tame in the energies of both fire and water in the human body.

Japanese Name: Shinbu-to
Chinese Name: Zhen Wu Tang
Scientific Name: Formula divinitatis nigrae

Common Brand Names

Ginger, Aconite, Hoelen & Peony Combination
Shinbu-to (Honso,* Tsumura*)
Shinbuto Formula 030 (Kampo Institute*)
Vital Energy (Qualiherb)
Vitality Combination (Sun Ten)
Zhen Wu Tang (Herbal Times, Lotus Classics, Qualiherb, Sun Ten)
(*Made in Japan)

Herbs Used to Make a Single Dose

Poria 4.0 g
Peony Root 3.0 g
White Atractylodis Rhizome 3.0 g
Ginger (fresh) 1.5 g
Aconite Tuber 0.5 g

Health Conditions Treated

Asthma, asthma in children, bronchitis, colds, and emphysema.

Who Should Use This Formula?

Weak patients with marked disturbance of metabolism and respiratory distress. Practitioners of Kampo medicine in Japan are especially likely to recommend this formula to persons with chronic viral infections such as hepatitis, herpes, and HIV, or autoimmune conditions such as multiple sclerosis, rheumatoid arthritis, and Sjögren's syndrome.

Consider This Formula If You Have Any of the Health Conditions Listed Above and Experience

Exhaustion, cold limbs, diarrhea without burning sensation in the anus, tremor, racing heart, and/or respiratory distress.

Energy Diagnosis

This formula is appropriate for an energy diagnosis of:

- Fifth Stage of Disease
- Yin deficiency
- *Ki* deficiency
- Cold in the interior energy layers of the body and energy deficiencies in all five organs

Explanation

The venerable herbalist Zhang Zhong-jing wrote, "When in the First Stage of Disease, sweating has been promoted and sweat issues but the disease does not resolve, the person still has heat effusion, and there are palpitations below the heart, dizzy head, generalized twitching, and the person is about to faint, True Warrior Formula cures."

Zhang Zhong-jing created this formula for a condition in which herbal treatment has enabled the body to successfully "sweat out" an infection, but the energy channels are depleted of *ki*. When there is a deficiency of energy, there is frequently an excess of fluid. The depletion of *ki* in the kidneys and digestive tract causes fluids to spill over into the flesh and skin, producing generalized swelling and body aches. Water ascending prevents "turbid" energy from descending, so the sense organs are veiled and thought is muddled. Water overwhelms the heart and causes palpitations, overwhelms the lungs and causes coughing, and overwhelms the intestines and causes diarrhea. All of these symptoms occur *after* the original infection has been overcome by the immune system.

Documentation

Today True Warrior Decoction is used to bolster the sympathetic nervous system to counteract the effects of anorexia and wasting. The sympathetic nervous system is the body's automatic control system for responding to environmental changes. On a cold day, the sympathetic nervous system ordinarily signals the brain that blood vessels in the skin, especially in the hands and feet, should be constricted to reduce the flow of blood to the skin and to reduce the loss of heat from the body. In the advanced stages of chronic disease, however, the sympathetic nervous system is unable to make fine adjustments in the control of the muscles controlling blood vessels. The result may be a feeling of cold, or a pooling of blood in the lower extremities depriving the brain of oxygen. Blood vessels that do not receive the sympathetic nervous system's signal to tighten also fail to circulate fluids. The result can be swollen feet, swollen ankles, swollen legs, and swollen hands.

The scientific research on True Warrior Decoction is preliminary, but laboratory experiments show that it reactivates tired adrenal glands.[1] The adrenaline these glands produce stimulates the sympathetic nervous system, and corrects the poor venous tone that causes coldness, palpitations, fainting, and swelling.

Uncaria Powder

Japanese Name: Choto-san
Chinese Name: Tian Ma Gou Teng Yin
Scientific Name: Pulvis uncariae

Common Brand Names

Choto-san (Honso,* Tsumura*)

Chinese- and American-made formulas that have the same effects and that contain the same herbs plus gastrodia powder include:

Gastrodia & Gambir Combination (Lotus Classics)
Gastrodia & Uncaria Combination (Sun Ten)
Gastrodia & Uncaria Formula (Chinese Classics, Golden Flower Chinese Herbs)

Gastrodia & Uncaria Wind Relief (Kan Traditionals)
Gastrodia Relieve Wind (Health Concerns)
Jian Ya (ProBotanixx)
Tian Ma Gou Teng Yin (Chinese Classics, Golden Flower Chinese Herbs, Herbal Times, Kan Traditionals, Lotus Classics, ProBotanixx, Qualiherb, Sun Ten)
Uncaria & Gastrodia (Qualiherb,)
(*Made in Japan)

Herbs Used to Make a Single Dose

Gypsum 5.0 g
Chen-Pi Peel 3.0 g
Sprouted Barley Seed 3.0 g
Pinellia Tuber 3.0 g
Poria 3.0 g
Ginseng 2.0 g
Ledebouriella Root 2.0 g
Licorice Root 1.0 g
Ginger (fresh) 1.0 g
Uncaria Ramulus ("Hooks") 3.0 g
Chrysanthemum Flowers 2.0 g

This formula uses the "hooks" that the stem of the uncaria plant grows to attach itself to trees.

Health Conditions Treated

Chronic headache and hypertension.

Who Should Use This Formula?

Strongly built persons with weak constitution in middle age, children with neurological disorders.

Consider This Formula If You Have Any of the Health Conditions Listed Above and Experience

Chronic headache, painful tension of shoulder and neck muscles, morning headache, feeling of heaviness in the head, feeling of uprising heat, ringing in the ears, and/or insomnia.

Energy Diagnosis

This formula is appropriate for an energy diagnosis of:

- Second Stage of Disease
- *Oketsu*
- Yang Symptoms
- *Ki* deficiency

Explanation

This formula, in both its Chinese and Japanese variations, is intended to treat a condition termed "liver-wind." In this syndrome the pent-up energies of emotion escape the body and cause sudden disturbances throughout the central nervous system. Liver-wind particularly affects the mental processes and sight. It also raises blood pressure.

Documentation

Kampo medicine uses gambir and gastrodia in many formulas for the treatment of seizures in children. Although the idea that aspartame (Nutra-Sweet) may trigger seizures is scientifically controversial, the pharmacological action of Uncaria Formula is especially well suited for preventing seizures, attention deficit, memory loss, or mood swings related to the consumption of aspartame, MSG, or processed foods.[1] A small-scale clinical study in Japan recently found that Uncaria Formula helps restore circulation to the brain in people who have transient ischemic attacks ("mini-strokes"), and also lowers total cholesterol.[2]

White Tiger Formula with Ginseng

In Japanese legend, Seiryu, the bluegreen dragon (who lent his name to *sho-seiryu-to*, Minor Bluegreen Dragon Formula) ruled the eastern sky. The eastern sky was the domain of spring. Seiryu gave power to new life, but he was not always the undisputed ruler of the eastern part of heaven. From time to time, a young tiger who descended from Orion's belt would spar with Seiryu. During these battles the dragon's fire and smoke became lightning and rain of spring storms. As the sun turned to summer, Dragon eventually tamed Tiger and as they fought less and less and the rains of spring came to an end. Dragon showed Tiger the virtues of containment as the rains were withheld from the summer sky. As Tiger learned the lessons of control, his mane became white. He thus earned the name, Byakko, or White Tiger. The White Tiger became the vessel of the energies of transformation, the ruler of the autumn season. White Tiger formula controlled the diseases of the autumn season: fever, thirst, sweating, and skin eruptions.

Japanese Name: Byakko-ka-ninjin-to
Chinese Name: Bai Hu Jia Ren Shen Tang
Scientific Name: Formula tigridis albi cum ginseng

Common Brand Names

Bai Hu Jai Ren Shen Tang (Lotus Classics, Qualiherb, Sun Ten)
Byakko-ka-ninjin-to (Honso,* Tsumura*)
Ginseng & Gypsum (Qualiherb)
Ginseng & Gypsum Combination (Lotus Classics, Sun Ten)
(*Made in Japan)

Herbs Used to Make a Single Dose

Gypsum 15.0 g

Anemarrhena Root 5.0 g
Licorice Root 2.0 g
Ginseng 1.5 g
Sticky Rice 8.0 g

Health Conditions Treated

Acne and eczema.

Who Should Use This Formula?

Physically active individual experiencing acute symptoms of the health conditions listed above.

Consider This Formula If You Have Any of the Health Conditions Listed Above and Experience

Feeling of heat in the entire body, fever, thirst, sweating, and/or skin eruptions.

Energy Diagnosis

This formula is appropriate for an energy diagnosis of:

- Third Stage of Disease
- Yang symptoms
- *Ki* excess

Explanation

In the symptom pattern this formula treats, an infection or energy imbalance has nearly conquered the outer three energy layers of the body. The body makes a last-ditch effort to overcome the pathogen by generating intense heat and high fever. The energy channels activated in the Third Stage of Disease carry heat to the head and face, so that there will be headache, redness in the face, and skin outbreaks especially on the face and shoulders. Because this heat is generated in the interior of the body, the alternating fever and chills found in the first two stages of disease are replaced by unremitting fever.

Documentation

The pharmacological action of White Tiger Formula with Ginseng is surprisingly simple. All of the ingredients except licorice and rice are either laxative or diuretic, stimulating bowel movement or urination. The herbs eliminate heat by expelling stool, which, being in the core of the body, contains considerable body heat. The herbs slow the pulse and reduce sweating by reducing the amount of fluid in the body, while helping the body conserve potassium.

These characteristics explain the traditional application of White Tiger Formula with Ginseng in treating febrile diseases and also explain its ability to relieve acne. Especially in adolescents, acne is associated with a buildup of testosterone. As the body uses testosterone it breaks it down into its constituent chemicals, the excess of which are excreted with stool. When there is constipation, however, stool remains in the body long enough for intestinal bacteria to reassemble the building blocks of testosterone for reabsorption into the bloodstream. White Tiger Formula with Ginseng stops this process.

Comparisons to Other Formulas

Five-Ingredient Powder with Poria may be taken with this formula when there is diarrhea, nausea, or vomiting.

Polyporus Formula may be more effective when there is scanty urination.

Tonify the Middle and Augument the *Qi* Formula may be a helpful addition when there are also kidney problems.

Part II

和漢薬

Introduction:

High-Class Medicine, Low-Class Medicine, Middle-Class Medicine

In its first thousand years of written history, Kampo medicine suffered an excess of innovation. The *Imperial Grace Formulary of the Tai Ping Era,* written in China between 982 and 992 A.D., contained 16,834 formulas. The *Ishimpo,* the great encyclopedia of Japanese herbal medicine presented to the Imperial Court in 984, required thirty volumes. The practical value of Kampo medicine was at risk of being obscured by the incessant presentation of new products, new ideas, and finer and finer distinctions of medical treatment.

The answer to information overload in the tenth century was found in three relatively slim volumes about Kampo medicine, the *Shen Nung*

Pen Ts'ao, or the *Pharmacopoeia of Heavenly Husbandry*. This herbal treatment manual presented 365 formulas, one for each day of the year, divided into three categories:

- 120 *Joyaku*, or Upper Class Medicines, remedies containing nourishment for an active life into old age. These medicines were intended to be taken every day over a period of years, and produced no unintended effects.

- 120 *Chuyuku*, or Middle Class Medicines, formulas intended to regenerate energy and keep the body in shape. These medicines would not produce side effects, but could not be used by everyone. They were only intended to address certain conditions of energy imbalance, and only intended to be taken as long as disease persisted.

- 125 *Shimoyaku*, or Low Class Medicines, combinations of herbs designed to treat serious illnesses. These medicines were only meant to be taken as long as acute symptoms persisted and were meant to taken under a physician's care.

Part 3 of this book is a listing of modern *Chuyuku*. The patent medicines listed here will not harm anyone who takes them in recommended dosages. They will correct energy imbalances that cause disease. They will not help everyone, however, and must be applied in accordance with assessment of *ki*, blood, fluids, and organ systems as shown by the checklists in Part 1.

Entries in Part 3 are organized in the same manner as Part 2. These are the various Japanese, Chinese, and English names under which the formula is sold in English-speaking countries. For each of the formulas listed in Part 3, you will find a complete listing of synonyms and brand names. Following the list of names are lists of the herbs the formula contains and medical conditions it treats.

Next is a "test question" that will allow you to decide whether the formula meets your unique health needs. Each formula treats a unique combination of symptoms. This combination of symptoms applies to more than one disease. You can use the scoring charts in Part 1 to make your own energy diagnosis and determine whether the formula is likely to treat the symptoms you experience. Then, if your physician has given you a diagnosis of one of the medical conditions listed for the formula, and you experience a *majority* of the symptoms the formula treats, the formula will be helpful in controlling your underlying health condition.

If your health condition matches the indications for the formula, it *will* help you. Sometimes, however, another formula will help you more. The final section of some entries lists other formulas that treat slight variations of symptoms that are treated with slight variations of the formula under another name.

Artemisia Formula

Japanese Name: Inchinko-to
Chinese Name: Yin Chen Hao Tang
Scientific Name: Formula artemisiae capillaris

Common Brand Names

Capillaris Combination (KPC Herbs, Lotus Classics, Qualiherb, Sun Ten)
Yin Chen Hao Tang (KPC Herbs, Lotus Classics, Qualiherb, Sun Ten)

Herbs Used to Make a Single Dose

Gardenia Fruit 3.0 g
Rhubarb Root 1.0 g
Artemisia Leaf 4.0 g

Health Conditions Treated

Hepatitis C.

Who Should Use This Formula?

Individuals with chronic hepatitis C who are capable of regular daily activities. This formula is especially suitable for persons with chronic hepatitis C or cirrhosis who do not have pain related to the disease. It is not recommended for children, pregnant women, or anyone who has a tendency for diarrhea.

Consider This Formula If You Have Any of the Health Conditions Listed Above and Experience

Nausea, constipation, and/or a feeling of fullness in the upper abdomen and the chest. Some people with this syndrome experience intermittent skin outbreaks, itch, dry mouth, or mouth sores.

Energy Diagnosis

This formula is appropriate for an energy diagnosis of:

- First Stage of Disease
- Stasis of fluids. *Ki* becomes congested in the middle layers of the body causing insufficient circulation of body fluids.

Augmented Restore the Spleen Decoction

In East Asian medicine, restoring the spleen refers to rejuvenating the energies of the digestive system. An augmented formula is especially fortified for difficult applications.

Japanese Name: Kami-kihi-to
Chinese Name: Jia Wei Gui Pi Tang
Latin Name: Formula lienalis angelicae compositae

Common Brand Names

Ginseng & Longan Combination Modified (Qualiherb, Sun Ten)
Jia Wei Gui Pi Tang (Qualiherb, Sun Ten)

Herbs Used to Make a Single Dose

Ginseng Root 3.0 g
White Atractylodis Root 3.0 g
Poria Mushroom 3.0 g
Astragalus Root 3.0 g
Dong Quai Root 2.0 g
Polygala Root 2.0 g
Bupleurum Root 3.0 g
Gardenia Fruit 2.0 g
Licorice Root 1.0 g
Saussurea Root 1.0 g
Jujube Fruit 2.0 g
Ginger (fresh) 1.0 g
Gardenia Fruit 3.0 g
Longan Fruit 3.0 g

Health Conditions Treated

Adult ADD/ADHD, anxiety, and insomnia.

Who Should Use This Formula?

Physically inactive or weak persons who experience restlessness, insomnia, or unexplained fear.

Consider This Formula If You Have Any of the Health Conditions Listed Above and Experience

Physical and psychic weakness, tendency for fear, and/or unexplained neurological symptoms (such as twitches, memory lapses, or fainting spells).

Energy Diagnosis

This formula is appropriate for an energy diagnosis of:

- Second Stage of Disease
- *Ki* neither excessive nor deficient

Comparisons to Other Formulas

Cinnamon, Dragon Bone, and Oyster Shell Formula may be more effective when there is no fever and predominant symptoms are fear and restlessness.

Coptis Antidote may be more effective when there is general nervousness or excitement, feeling of heat in the whole body, and widespread muscle tension.

Ten-Significant Tonic Formula may be more effective if there is coldness in hands and feet, tendency for fever, and/or irritability.

Bupleurum and Cinnamon Formula

Japanese Name: Saiko-keishi-to
Chinese Name: Chai Hu Gui Zhi Tang
Scientific Name: Formula cinnamomi et bupleuri

Common Brand Names

Bupleurum & Cinnamon Combination (KPC Herbs, Lotus Classics, Qualiherb, Sun Ten)

Bupleurum & Cinnamon Formula (Golden Flower Chinese Herbs)

Chai Hu Gui Zhi Tang (Golden Flower Chinese Herbs, Health

Concerns, Honso,* KPC Herbs, Lotus Classics, Qualiherb, Sun Ten)
Ease 2 (Health Concerns)
Kampo4Cold/Flu Cinnamon Formula (Honso*)
Saiko-keishi-to (Honso,* Tsumura*)
Saikokeishito Formula 015 (Kampo Institute*)
(* Made in Japan)

Herbs Used to Make a Single Dose

Bupleurum Root 5.0 g
Pinellia Tuber 4.0 g
Ginseng Root 2.0 g
Jujube Fruit 2.0 g
Licorice Root 2.0 g
Ginger (fresh) 1.0 g
Scutellaria Root 2.0 g
Cinnamon Bark 2.0 g
Peony Root 2.0 g

Health Conditions Treated

Colds, gallbladder irritation, gallstones, hepatitis, pancreatitis, pneumonia, and tuberculosis of the lungs.

Who Should Use This Formula?

Physically active individuals who are not incapacitated by disease.

Consider This Formula If You Have Any of the Health Conditions Listed Above and Experience

Fever, mild headache, chills, loss of appetite, joint pain, pain in the area above the stomach, restlessness, fear, insomnia, and/or tenderness on the right side of the abdomen.

Energy Diagnosis

This formula is appropriate for an energy diagnosis of:

- Second Stage of Disease
- *Ki* deficiency

Bupleurum plus Dragon Bone and Oyster Shell Formula

Japanese Name: Saiko-ka-ryukotsu-borei-to
Chinese Name: Chai Hu Jia Long Gu Mu Li Tang
Scientific Name: Formula bupleuri cum ostrea et osse fossile

Common Brand Names

Chai Hu Long Gu Mu Li Wan (Herbal Times)
Saiko-ka-ryukotsu-borei-to (Honso,* Tsumura*)
(*Made in Japan)

Herbs Used to Make a Single Dose

Bupleurum Root 5.0
Scutellaria Root 2.5 g
Pinellia Tuber 4.0 g
Cinnamon Bark 3.0 g
Oyster Shell 2.5 g
Poria Mushroom 3.0 g
Jujube Fruit 2.5 g
Ginseng Root 2.5 g
Dragon Bone (fossilized mastodon bone) 2.5 g
Ginger (fresh) 1.0 g

Health Conditions Treated

Crying fits of children at night, hypertension, hysteria, mood swings, excessive urination, and tachycardia (especially when sensitive to emotional stress). Recent research suggests formula may stop hardening of the arteries in people who have high cholesterol.

Who Should Use This Formula?

Relatively strong persons who are not incapacitated by symptoms.

Consider This Formula If You Have Any of the Health Conditions Listed Above and Experience

Restlessness, fear, insomnia, heavy feeling in the head, painful tension of shoulder and neck muscles, palpitations, fast pulse, emotional instability, and/or extrasystoles (extra heart beats).

Energy Diagnosis

This formula is appropriate for an energy diagnosis of:

- Second Stage of Disease
- *Ki* excess

Comparisons with Other Formulas

Cinnamon, Dragon Bone, and Oyster Shell Formula may be more effective when there is no racing pulse.

Coptis Antidote may be a helpful addition to the formula when primary symptoms of concern are mood swings and insomnia.

Bupleurum, Cinnamon, and Ginger Formula

Japanese Name: Saiko-keishi-kankyo-to
Chinese Name: Chai Hu Gui Zhi Gan Jiang Tang
Scientific Name: Formula zingiberis siccati cinnamomi bupleuri

Common Brand Names

Bupleurum, Cinnamon Twig, and Ginger Combination (KPC Herbs)
Chai Hu Gui Zhi Gan Jiang Tang (KPC Herbs)

Herbs Used to Make a Single Dose

Bupleurum Root 6.0 g
Scutellaria Root 3.0 g
Tricosanthis Root 3.0 g
Cinnamon Bark 3.0 g
Oyster Shell 3.0 g
Licorice Root 2.0 g
Ginger (dried) 2.0 g

Health Conditions Treated

Insomnia, discomforts of menopause, and fatigue caused by chronic bronchitis, hepatitis, and nephritis.

Who Should Use This Formula?

Persons with a weak constitution and "cold" symptoms (sensitivity to the cold, pale complexion, cold hands or feet, etc.).

Consider This Formula If You Have Any of the Health Conditions Listed Above and Experience

Exhaustion, racing heart, shortness of breath, insomnia, pain below the stomach or under the rib cage, chills, fever, nightsweats, and/or thirst.

Energy Diagnosis

This formula is appropriate for an energy diagnosis of:

- Second Stage of Disease
- Stasis of fluids
- Imbalance of *ki*

Comparisons to Other Formulas

Tonify the Middle and Augment the *Qi* Formula may be more effective when there is high fever.

Calm the Middle Powder

Japanese Name: Anchu-san
Chinese Name: An Zhong San
Scientific Name: Pulvis liberationis abdominis

Common Brand Names

An Zhong San (KPC Herbs, Lotus Classics, Qualiherb, Sun Ten)
Anchu-san (Honso,* Tsumura*)
Cardamon & Fennel (Qualiherb)
Cardamon & Fennel Formula (Sun Ten)
Fennel & Galanga Formula (KPC Herbs, Lotus Classics)
(* Made in Japan)

Herbs Used to Make a Single Dose

Cinnamon Bark 4.0 g
Corydalis Tuber 3.0 g
Oyster Shell 3.0 g
Fennel Seed 1.5 g
Licorice Root 1.0 g

Cardamom Seed 1.0 g
Galangal Root 0.5 g

Health Conditions Treated

Gastritis.

Who Should Use This Formula?

Individuals with progressive chronic diseases of any kind who have a long-term tendency to poor appetite, weak abdominal muscles, and/or sloshing sounds in the upper stomach after eating.

Consider This Formula If You Have Any of the Health Conditions Listed Above and Experience

Mild abdominal pain, stomach pain, belching, nausea, vomiting, loss of appetite, and/or stomach pain in stressful-situations.

Energy Diagnosis

This formula is appropriate for an energy diagnosis of:

- Second Stage of Disease
- Stasis of *ki* and body fluids

Comparisons with Other Formulas

Calm the Stomach Powder offers more effective relief of gas.

Calm the Stomach and Poria Formula

Japanese Name: Irei-to
Chinese Name: Wei Ling Tang
Scientific Name: Formula poria stomachi

Common Brand Names

Magnolia & Hoelen Combination (KPC Herbs, Lotus Classics, Qualiherb)

Wei Ling Tang (KPC Herbs, Lotus Classics, Qualiherb)

Herbs Used to Make a Single Dose

Magnolia Bark 2.5 g
White Atractylodis Rhizome 2.5 g
Alisma Rhizome 2.5 g
Polyporus Mushroom 2.5 g
Bitter Orange Peel 2.5 g
White Atractylodis Rhizome 2.5 g
Poria Mushroom 2.5 g
Cinnamon Bark 2.0 g
Ginger (fresh) 1.5 g
Jujube Fruit 1.5 g
Licorice Root 1.0 g

Health Conditions Treated

Diarrhea.

Who Should Use This Formula?

Physically active, vigorous individuals who experience acute symptoms of diarrhea, especially after exercise in heat and taking lots of liquids.

Consider This Formula If You Have Any of the Health Conditions Listed Above and Experience

Watery diarrhea, sloshing sounds in digestive tract after eating, bloating, gas, vomiting, thirst, scanty urine, loss of appetite, and/or mild abdominal pain.

Energy Diagnosis

This formula is appropriate for an energy diagnosis of:

- Second Stage of Disease
- *Ki* deficiency
- Stasis of fluids

Comparisons to Other Formulas

Calm the Stomach Powder may be more effective when there is bloating and gas, but not diarrhea.

Calm the Stomach Powder

Japanese Name: Heii-san
Chinese Name: Ping Wei San
Scientific Name: Pulvis ad auxilium stomachi

Common Brand Names

Magnolia & Ginger (Qualiherb)
Magnolia & Ginger Formula (KPC Herbs, Lotus Classics, Sun Ten)
Ping Wei San (Health Concerns, KPC Herbs, Lotus Classics, Qualiherb, Sun Ten)
Stomach Tabs (Health Concerns)

Herbs Used to Make a Single Dose

White Atractylodis Rhizome 4.0 g
Magnolia Bark 3.0 g
Bitter Orange Peel 3.0 g
Jujube Fruit 2.0 g
Licorice Root 1.0 g

Ginger (fresh) 0.5 g

Chinese versions of this formula omit ginger and jujube.

Health Conditions Treated

Gastritis and peptic ulcer.

Who Should Use This Formula?

Persons whose daily routine is not compromised by disease.

Warning: This formula should not be taken by women in the third trimester of pregnancy. It has been known to induce labor.

Consider This Formula If You Have Any of the Health Conditions Listed Above and Experience

Accumulation of fluid in the stomach, bloating, gas, loss of appetite, "stomach rumbles," and/or diarrhea.

Energy Diagnosis

This formula is appropriate for an energy diagnosis:

- Second Stage of Disease
- Yang deficiency
- *Ki* deficiency

Comparisons to Other Formulas

Calm the Middle Powder may be more effective when there is chronic pain in the upper abdomen, there is no sound of fluctuating liquid in the digestive tract, and heartburn is a especially troublesome symptom.

Ginseng Formula may be more effective when there is *ki* deficiency and there is no bloating or gas.

Cimicifuga and Kudzu Formula

(This formula is also known as Black Cohosh and Kudzu Formula.)

Japanese Name: Shoma-kakkon-to
Chinese Name: Sheng Ma Ge Gen Tang
Scientific Name: Formula puerariae et cimicifugae

Common Brand Names

Cimicifuga & Pueraria Combination (KPC Herbs, Lotus Classics, Qualiherb, Sun Ten)
Sheng Ma Ge Gen Tang (KPC Herbs, Lotus Classics, Qualiherb, Sun Ten)

Herbs Used to Make a Single Dose

Kudzu Root 5.0 g
Peony Root 3.0 g
Black Cohosh 2.0 g
Licorice Root 1.5 g
Ginger (fresh) 0.5 g

Health Conditions Treated

Allergic reactions of the skin, contact dermatitis, herpes, hives, and measles.

Who Should Use This Formula?

Anyone experiencing an acute skin outbreak.

Consider This Formula If You Have Any of the Health Conditions Listed Above and Experience

Skin outbreaks of various kinds, pain throughout the body, headache, and/or fever and chills.

Energy Diagnosis

This formula is appropriate for an energy diagnosis of:

- First Stage of Disease
- *Ki* neither deficient nor excessive

Cinnamon, Aconite, and Atractylodis Formula

Japanese Name: Keishi-ka-jutsubu-to
Chinese Name: Gui Zhi Jia Fu Zi Bai Zhu Tang
Latin Name: Formula cinnamomi cum rehi et paeonia

Common Brand Names

Cinnamon, Aconite, and Ginger Combination (Brion)
Keishi-ka-jutsubu-to (Honso,* Tsumura*)
(* Made in Japan)

Herbs Used to Make a Single Dose

Peony Root 6.0 g
Cinnamon Bark 4.0 g
Jujube Fruit 4.0 g
Ginger (fresh) 4.0 g
Licorice Root 2.0 g
White Atractylodis Root 1.0 g
Aconite Tuber 0.5

Health Conditions Treated

Neuralgia, osteoarthritis, and rheumatoid arthritis.

Who Should Use This Formula?

Physically weak patients with mobility problems.

Consider This Formula If You Have Any of the Health Conditions Listed Above and Experience

Reduced mobility of joints, swollen joints, and/or muscle pain, all aggravated by cold. From time to time, persons with this syndrome may also experience mild fever, morning stiffness, or scanty urination.

Energy Diagnosis

This formula is appropriate for an energy diagnosis of:

- Fourth Stage of Disease
- *Ki* deficiency
- Stasis of fluids

Cinnamon and Ginseng Formula

Japanese Name: Keishi-ninjin-to
Chinese Name: Gui Zhi Ren Shen Tang
Scientific Name: Formula ginseng et cinnamomi

Common Brand Names

Cinnamon & Ginseng Combination (KPC Herbs)
Gui Zhi Ren Shen Tang (KPC Herbs)
Keishininjinto Formula 013 (Kampo Institute*)
(*Made in Japan)

Herbs Used to Make a Single Dose

Cinnamon Bark 4.0 g
Licorice Root 3.0 g

White Atractylodis Root 3.0g
Ginseng Root 3.0 g
Ginger (dried) 2.0 g

Health Conditions Treated

Colds and flu accompanied by burning diarrhea or chronic headache

Who Should Use This Formula?

Persons in a relatively weakened state, forced to withdraw from daily activities by colds or flu.

Consider This Formula If You Have Any of the Health Conditions Listed Above and Experience

Pale complexion but occasional hot flashes causing redness in the face, fever in the head and face but cold hands and feet, rumbling sounds in the stomach, hypersensitivity to cold, and/or tension around the anus during defecation.

Energy Diagnosis

This formula is appropriate for an energy diagnosis of:

- Fourth Stage of Disease
- *Ki* deficiency
- Yin excess

Cinnamon and Peony Formula

Japanese Name: Keishi-ka-shakuyaku-to
Chinese Name: Gui Zhi Shao Yao Tang
Scientific Name: Formula cinnamomi cum paeonia

Common Brand Names

Cinnamon & Peony Combination (KPC Herbs, Lotus Classics, Qualiherb, Sun Ten)

Gui Zhi Jia Shao Yao Tang (KPC Herbs, Lotus Classics, Qualiherb, Sun Ten)

Herbs Used to Make a Single Dose

Peony Root 6.0 g
Cinnamon Bark 4.0 g
Jujube Fruit 4.0 g
Licorice Root 2.0 g
Ginger (fresh) 1.0 g

Health Conditions Treated

Chronic constipation, colitis, food poisoning, irritable bowel syndrome, and kidney stones.

Who Should Use This Formula?

Persons whose physical activities are curtailed by illness.

Consider This Formula If You Have Any of the Health Conditions Listed Above and Experience

Abdominal pain, diarrhea, pain during defecation, feeling of cold in the abdomen, bloating and gas, and/or spasms of the abdominal muscles and muscles surrounding the anal sphincter.

Energy Diagnosis

This formula is appropriate for an energy diagnosis of:

- Fourth Stage of Disease
- *Ki* deficiency
- Yin excess

Cinnamon and Poria Pill

Japanese Name: Keishi-bukuryo-gan
Chinese Name: Gui Zhi Fu Ling Wan
Scientific Name: Pilulae poria et cinnamomi

Common Brand Names

Cinnamon & Hoelen Formula (KPC Herbs, Lotus Classics, Sun Ten)
Cinnamon & Poria Formula (Golden Flower Chinese Herbs)
Gui Zhi Fu Ling Wan (Golden Flower Chinese Herbs, Herbal Times, Honso,* Kan Herbals, KPC Herbs, Lotus Classics, Sun Ten)
Kampo4Women MonthlyEase (Honso*)
Keishi-bukuryo-gan (Honso,* Tsumura*)
Keishibukuryogan Formula 018 (Kampo Institute*)
Women's Chamber (Kan Herbals)
(*Made In Japan)

Herbs Used to Make a Single Dose

Cinnamon Bark 3.0 g
Peony Root 3.0 g
Peach Seed 3.0 g
Poria Mushroom 3.0 g
Moutan Root 3.0 g

Health Conditions Treated

Bruises after trauma, endometriosis, discomforts of menopause, missed or scanty periods, pelvic inflammatory disease, swollen testicles, and pain after vasectomy.

Who Should Use This Formula?

Persons whose physical activities are not impeded by disease.

Consider This Formula If You Have Any of the Health Conditions Listed Above and Experience

Feeling of uprising heat, red face, headache, tension in the neck and shoulders, cold feet, and/or sensitivity to cold.

Energy Diagnosis

This formula is appropriate for an energy diagnosis of:

- Second Stage of Disease
- Oketsu

Coptis Formula

Japanese Name: Oren-to
Chinese Name: Huang Lian Tang
Latin Name: Formula coptidis

Common Brand Names

Huang Lian Tang (KPC Herbs, Sun Ten)
Coptis Combination (KPC Herbs, Sun Ten)

Herbs Used to Make a Single Dose

Pinellia Tuber 6.0 g
Coptis Rhizome 3.0 g
Licorice Root 3.0g
Cinnamon Bark 3.0 g
Jujube Fruit 3.0 g
Ginseng Root 3.0 g
Ginger (fresh) 3.0 g

Health Conditions Treated

Gastroenteritis, peptic ulcers, stomatitis (mouth sores), and unusual sensitivity to cold.

Who Should Use This Formula?

Physically active individuals with a tendency to digestive complaints.

Consider This Formula If You Have Any of the Health Conditions Listed Above and Experience

Heat in the upper part of the body and cold in the lower part of the body, frequent stomach upset which is worse under conditions of emotional stress, restlessness, headache, and/or mild fever.

Energy Diagnosis

This formula is appropriate for an energy diagnosis of:

- Second Stage of Disease
- *Ki* deficiency

Comparisons to Other Formulas

Bupleurum and Cinnamon Formula offers more effective relief when there is abdominal tension.

Ginseng Formula is more effective when symptoms include cold hands and feet.

Cyperus and Perilla Powder

Japanese Name: Koso-san
Chinese Name: Xiang Su San
Scientific Name: Pulvis perillae et cyperi

Common Brand Names

Xiang Su San (KPC Herbs, Lotus Classics, Qualiherb, Sun Ten)

Cyperus & Perilla Formula (KPC Herbs, Lotus Classics, Qualiherb, Sun Ten)

Koso-san (Honso,* Tsumura*)

(* Made in Japan)

Herbs Used to Make a Single Dose

Cyperus Rhizome 4.0 g

Perilla Leaf 2.0 g

Bitter Orange Peel 2.0 g

Licorice Root 1.5

Ginger (fresh) 1.0 g

Health Conditions Treated

Hives, especially when due to an allergic reaction to fish, shellfish, or meat; initial stages of influenza; and discomforts of menopause.

Who Should Use This Formula?

Physically vigorous persons experiencing acute symptoms of disease.

Consider This Formula If You Have Any of the Health Conditions Listed Above and Experience

Blocked nose, headache, nausea, vomiting, bloating, depression, loss of appetite, nervousness, insomnia, and/or restlessness.

Energy Diagnosis

This formula is appropriate for an energy diagnosis of:

- First Stage of Disease
- *Ki* deficiency

Dong Quai Rejuvenation Formula

This formula is also known as Dong Quai (or Tang-kuei) Decoction to Construct the Middle.

Japanese Name: Toki-kenchu-to
Chinese Name: Dang Gui Jian Zhong Tang
Scientific Name: Formula salubritatis abdominis angelicae

Common Brand Names

Dang Gui & Cinnamon & Peony (Qualiherb)
Dang Gui Jian Zhong Tang (Qualiherb, Sun Ten)
Tang-kuei, Cinnamon, & Peony Combination (Sun Ten)

Herbs Used to Make a Single Dose

Peony Root 5.0 g
Cinnamon Bark 4.0 g
Jujube Fruit 4.0 g
Dong Quai Root 4.0 g
Licorice Root 2.0 g
Ginger (fresh) 1.0 g

Health Conditions Treated

Hemorrhoids.

Who Should Use This Formula?

Women, especially after childbirth.

Consider This Formula If You Have Any of the Health Conditions Listed Above and Experience

Anal prolapse, fatigue, pale complexion, cold hands and feet, abdominal pain, bleeding hemorrhoids, and/or freckles or age spots.

Energy Diagnosis

This formula is appropriate for an energy diagnosis of:

- Fourth Stage of Disease
- *Ki* deficiency
- Yin excess

Comparisons to Other Formulas

Astragalus Formula is a useful addition when there is also eczema.

Cinnamon and Peony Formula is a useful addition when there is also diarrhea.

Ephedra, Asiasarum, and Prepared Aconite Formula

Japanese Name: Mao-bushi-sashin-to
Chinese Name: M Ma Huang Fu Zi Xi Xin Tang
Scientific Name: Formula ephedrae cum aconiti et asiasari

Common Brand Names

Ma Huang & Asarum Combination (Sun Ten)
Ma Huang & Asarum (Qualiherb)
Ma Huang Fu Zi Xi Xin Tang (Qualiherb, Sun Tang)
Herbs Used to Make a Single Dose
Ephedra Leaf 4.0 g

Asiasarum (Asarum) Root 5.0 g
Aconite Tuber 1.0 g

Health Conditions Treated

Nasal allergy (especially to cedar pollen), colds, laryngitis, chronic coughing or wheezing, and tooth pain when drinking cold drinks.

Who Should Use This Formula?

Older persons with a marked susceptibility to the cold, or younger persons who have frequent colds.

Consider This Formula If You Have Any of the Health Conditions Listed Above and Experience

Sensitivity to cold, fatigue, slow pulse, headache, cough, runny nose, cold hands and feet, and/or weak immune system.

Energy Diagnosis

This formula is appropriate for an energy diagnosis of:

- Second Stage of Disease
- Yin deficiency
- *Ki* neither deficient nor excessive

Evodia Formula

Japanese Name: Goshuyu-to
Chinese Name: Wu Zhu Yu Tang
Scientific Name: Formula evodiae

Common Brand Names

Evodia Combination (KPC Herbs, Lotus Classics, Qualiherb, Sun Ten)
Goshuyuto Formula 020 (Kampo Institute*)
Go-shuyu-to (Honso,* Tsumura)
Wu Zhu Yu Tang (KPC Herbs, Lotus Classics, Qualiherb, Sun Ten)
(* Made in Japan)

Herbs Used to Make a Single Dose

Jujube Fruit 4.0 g
Evodia Fruit 3.0 g
Ginseng Root 2.0 g
Ginger (fresh) 1.5 g

Health Conditions Treated

Migraine.

Who Should Use This Formula?

Physically weak individuals with marked sensitivity to cold.

Consider This Formula If You Have Any of the Health Conditions Listed Above and Experience

Painful tension of the shoulder and neck muscles, vomiting, bloating, stomach rumbles, feeling of heaviness in the abdomen, and/or cold hands and feet.

Energy Diagnosis

This formula is appropriate for an energy diagnosis of:

- Fourth Stage of Disease
- *Ki* deficiency (due to nutritional deficiency)

Comparisons with Other Formulas

Cinnamon and Ginseng Formula may be more effective when there is a tendency for diarrhea.

Uncaria Powder is a helpful addition to this formula when emotional instability is a symptom of primary concern.

Five Tiger Formula

Japanese Name: Goko-to
Chinese Name: Wu Hu Tang
Scientific Name: Formula quinque-tigrium

Common Brand Names

Gypsum & Apricot Seed Combination (Brion Herbs)
Wu Hu Tang (Brion Herbs)

Herbs Used to Make a Single Dose

Gypsum 10.0 g
Peach Seed 4.0 g
Ephedra Leaf 4.0 g
Mulberry Bark 3.0 g
Licorice Root 2.0 g

Health Conditions Treated

Bronchial asthma, bronchitis, bronchial spasm, and common cold.

Who Should Use This Formula?

Children who have not yet required bed rest for respiratory symptoms.

Consider This Formula If You Have Any of the Health Conditions Listed Above and Experience

Shortness of breath, wheezing, severe attacks of coughing, thirst, sweating, and/or heavy phlegm.

Energy Diagnosis

This formula is appropriate for an energy diagnosis of:

- Second Stage of Disease
- *Ki* imbalance

Comparisons to Other Formulas

Japanese Lily formula may be added to relieve lump in the throat.

Five-Accumulation Powder

In Kampo, the five accumulations are blood, cold, dampness, energy (*qi*), and phlegm.

Japanese Name: Goshaku-san
Chinese Name: Wu Ji San
Scientific Name: Pulvis quinque-hystericorum

Common Brand Names

Dang Gui & Magnolia (Qualiherb)
Tangkuei & Magnolia Five Formula (KPC Herbs, Lotus Classics)
Tang-kuei & Magnolia Formula (Sun Ten)
Wu Ji San (KPC Herbs, Lotus Classics, Qualiherb, Sun Ten)

Herbs Used to Make a Single Dose

White Atractylodis Rhizome 3.0 g
Bitter Orange Peel 2.0 g
Dong Quai Root 2.0 g
Pinellia Tuber 2.0 g
Poria Mushroom 2.0 g

Licorice Root 1.0 g
Platycodon Root 1.0 g
Bitter Orange Fruit 1.0 g
Cinnamon Bark 1.0 g
Magnolia Bark 1.0 g
Peony Root 1.0 g
Ginger (fresh) 1.0 g
Ligusticum Root 1.0 g
Jujube Fruit 1.0 g
Dong Quai Root 1.0 g
Ephedra Leaf 1.0 g

Health Conditions Treated

Anemia, lower back pain, myalgia, and menstrual irregularities (missed or scanty periods, or menstrus containing pus).

Who Should Use This Formula?

Persons who are not underweight and who are have well-developed muscles.

Consider This Formula If You Have Any of the Health Conditions Listed Above and Experience

Pain in the lower abdomen or pelvis, muscle pain, chronic rheumatoid arthritis, headache, and/or heat in the upper part of the body with cold in the lower part of the body.

Energy Diagnosis

This formula is appropriate for an energy diagnosis of:

- Fourth Stage of Disease
- *Ki* neither deficient nor excessive
- Stasis of fluids

Five-Ingredient Powder for Painful Urinary Dysfunction

Japanese Name: Gorin-san
Chinese Name: Wu Lin San
Scientific Name: Pulvis qinque medicamentorum ad tractum urogenitalem.

Common Brand Names

Gardenia & Hoelen Formula (KPC Herbs, Lotus Classics, Qualiherb, Sun Ten)
Wu Lin San (KPC Herbs, Lotus Classics, Qualiherb, Sun Ten)

Herbs Used to Make a Single Dose

Poria Mushroom 6.0 g
Scutellaria Root 3.0 g
Licorice Root 3.0 g
Rehmannia Root 3.0 g
Psyllium Seed 3.0 g
Alisma Rhizome 3.0 g
Dong Quai Root 3.0 g
Akebia Stem 3.0 g
Gardenia Fruit 2.0 g
Peony Root 2.0 g
Kadinum (medicinal clay) 3.0 g

Health Conditions Treated

Bladder stones, irritable bladder, prostate inflammation, and urinary-tract infections.

Who Should Use This Formula?

Physically inactive persons who are not underweight.

Consider This Formula If You Have Any of the Health Conditions Listed Above and Experience

Pain during urination, weak stream of dark-colored urine, chronic infection of the urinary tract, and/or tendency to be sensitive to cold.

Energy Diagnosis

This formula is appropriate for an energy diagnosis of:

- Third Stage of Disease
- Stasis of fluids
- *Ki* neither deficient nor excessive

Comparisons to Other Formulas

Dong Quai and Gentian Formula may be more effective when emotional instability is a symptom of concern.

Polyporus Formula may be taken with this formula to relieve mild symptoms of inflammation and thirst.

Forsythia and Japanese Mint Formula

Japanese Name: Keigai-rengyo-to
Chinese Name: Jing Jie Lian Qiao Tang
Scientific Name: Formula forsythiae et schizonepetae

Common Brand Names

Jing Jie Lian Qiao Tang (KPC Herbs, Lotus Classics, Qualiherb, Sun Ten)

Schizonepeta & Forsythia Combination (KPC Herbs, Lotus Classics, Qualiherb, Sun Ten)

Herbs Used to Make a Single Dose

Scutellaria Root 1.5 g
Phellodendron Bark 1.5 g
Coptis Rhizome 1.5 g
Platycodon Root 1.5 g
Bitter Orange Fruit 1.5 g
Japanese Mint (Schizonepeta) Leaf 1.5 g
Bupleurum Root 1.5 g
Gardenia Fruit 1.5 g
Rehmannia Root 1.5 g
Peony Root 1.5 g
Ligusticum Root 1.5 g
Dong Quai Root 1.5 g
Mint Leaf and Stem 1.5 g
White Atractylodis Rhizome 1.5 g
Ledebouriella Root 1.5 g
Forsythia Fruit 1.5 g
Licorice Root 1.0 g

Health Conditions Treated

Acne, ear infections, eczema, hay fever, sinusitis, sore throat, and tonsillitis.

Who Should Use This Formula?

Physically active persons who have a tendency for skin outbreaks or upper respiratory infections.

Consider This Formula If You Have Any of the Health Conditions Listed Above and Experience

Skin outbreaks (acne, lumps, nodules, ulcer); pallor; sweaty palms and feet; and/or muscle tension.

Energy Diagnosis

This formula is appropriate for an energy diagnosis of:

- Second Stage of Disease
- *Ki* neither deficient nor excessive

Four-Gentleman Formula

Japanese Name: Shikunshi-to
Chinese Name: Si Jun Zi Tang
Scientific Name: Formula quadrorum medicamentorum nobilis

Common Brand Names

Astra 8 (Health Concerns)
Four Major Herb (Qualiherb)
Major Four Herb Combination (KPC Herbs, Lotus Classics, Sun Ten)
Shikunshi-to (Honso,* Tsumura*)
Si Jun Zi Tang (Health Concerns, KPC Herbs, Lotus Classics, Qualiherb, Sun Ten)
(*Made in Japan)

Herbs Used to Make a Single Dose

White Atractylodis Rhizome 4.0 g
Ginseng Root 4.0 g
Poria Mushroom 4.0 g
Licorice Root 1.0 g

Many Japanese versions of this formula also add:

Ginger (fresh) 1.0 g
Jujube Fruit 1.0 g

Health Conditions Treated

Exhaustion due to chronic disease, gastritis, gastric and duodenal ulcers, and disturbance of the digestive system due to surgery.

Who Should Use This Formula?

Physically weak individuals with disturbances of the digestive system.

Consider This Formula If You Have Any of the Health Conditions Listed Above and Experience

Fatigue, pale complexion, loss of appetite, nausea, vomiting, bloating, diarrhea, "stomach rumbles," and/or weak abdominal muscles.

Energy Diagnosis

This formula is appropriate for an energy diagnosis of:

- Fourth Stage of Disease
- Severe *ki* deficiency

Four-Substance Formula

Japanese Name: Shimotsu-to
Chinese Name: Si Wu Tang
Scientific Name: Formula quadrorum medicamentorum

Common Brand Names

Angelica Restorative Formula (Kan Traditionals)
Tangkuei 4 Combination (KPC Herbs)
Dang Gui 4 (Qualiherb)
Tang-kuei Four Combination (Sun Ten)
Bend Bamboo (Three Treasures)
Brighten the Eyes (Three Treasures)

Shikunshi-to (Honso,* Tsumura*)
(* Made in Japan)

Herbs Used to Make a Single Dose

Rehmannia Root 3.0 g
Peony Root 3.0 g
Ligusticum Rhizome 3.0 g
Dong Quai Root 3.0 g

Health Conditions Treated

Age spots, dysmenorrhea, infertility, hypertension, and discomforts of menopause.

Who Should Use This Formula?

Physically weakened individuals who cannot fully pursue daily life activities due to disease.

Consider This Formula If You Have Any of the Health Conditions Listed Above and Experience

Unusual sensitivity to cold, pale complexion, dry skin, and/or wrinkles.

Energy Diagnosis

This formula is appropriate for an energy diagnosis of:

- Fourth Stage of Disease
- *Oketsu*
- *Ki* deficiency

Comparisons to Other Formulas

Dong Quai and Peony Formula may be a helpful addition to this formula if there is swelling anywhere in the body, or recurrent abdominal pain.

Ginseng Formula

Japanese Name: Ninjin-to
Chinese Name: Ren Shen Tang
Scientific Name: Formula ginseng

Common Brand Names

Ginseng & Ginger Combination (Sun Ten)
Ninjinto Formula 022 (Kampo Institute*)
Ren Shen Tang (Sun Ten)
(* Made in Japan)

Herbs Used to Make a Single Dose

Ginseng Root 3.0 g
Ginger (dried) 3.0 g
Licorice Root 3.0 g
White Atractylodis Rhizome 3.0 g

Health Conditions Treated

Gastritis, stomach spasms, and morning sickness.

Who Should Use This Formula?

Physically weak persons with marked sensitivity to cold.

Consider This Formula If You Have Any of the Health Conditions Listed Above and Experience

Physical and emotional exhaustion, heavy feeling in the stomach, diarrhea, excessive urination, excessive salivation, markedly loose abdominal muscles, and/or "stomach rumbles."

Energy Diagnosis

This formula is appropriate for an energy diagnosis of:

- Fourth Stage of Disease
- *Ki* deficiency

Comparisons to Other Formulas

Evodia Formula may be more effective if headache and vomiting are primary symptoms of concern.

Cinnamon and Ginseng Formula may be more effective if headache and hot flashes are primary symptoms of concern.

Great Ledebouriella Formula

Japanese Name: Dai-bofu-to
Chinese Name: Da Fang Feng Tang
Scientific Name: Formula ledebouriellae major

Common Brand Names

Da Fang Feng Tang (KPC Herbs, Sun Ten)
Major Siler Combination (KPC Herbs, Sun Ten)

Herbs Used to Make a Single Dose

Astragalus Root 3.0 g
Ledebouriella Root 3.0 g
Ginseng Root 1.5 g
Rehmannia Root 3.0 g
Ligusticum Root 2.0 g
Notopterygium Rhizome 1.5 g
Peony Root 3.0 g
Licorice Root 1.5 g
Eucommia Bark 3.0 g
White Atractylodis Rhizome 3.0 g

Achyranthis Root 1.5 g
Ginger (dried) 1.0 g
Dong Quai Root 3.0 g
Jujube Fruit 1.5 g
Aconite Tuber 1.0 g

Health Conditions Treated

Osteoarthritis, rheumatoid arthritis of the legs and feet, gout, and obesity.

Who Should Use This Formula?

Physically weak persons of pale complexion.

Consider This Formula If You Have Any of the Health Conditions Listed Above and Experience

Weakness or atrophy of leg muscles. This formula originally was prescribed for "dysenteric wind," a condition in which the legs are so painful and weakened after an intestinal condition that it is very difficult to walk.

Energy Diagnosis

This formula is appropriate for an energy diagnosis of:

- Fourth Stage of Disease
- *Oketsu*

Comparisons to Other Formulas

Cinnamon, Aconite, and Atractylodis Formula may be added to relieve cramps.

Guide Out the Red Powder

This formula guides heat away from the heart, which Kampo medicine associates with the color red. It also treats "red" symptoms, such as red face, red tongue, and sores in the mouth.

Japanese Name: Do-seki-san
Chinese Name: Dao Chi San
Scientific Name: Formula rehmanniae et akebiae

Common Brand Names

Dao Chi San (KPC Herbs, Lotus Classics, Sun Ten)
Rehmannia & Lopatherum Formula (Sun Ten)
Rehmannia Akebia Formula (KPC Herbs, Lotus Classics)

Herbs Used to Make a Single Dose

Rehmannia Root 5.0 g
Mu Tan Caulis 3.0 g
Lophatherum Leaf 3.0 g
Licorice Root Tips 3.0 g

Health Conditions Treated

Nightmares in children, mouth sores, and urinary tract infections.

Who Should Use This Formula?

Children suffering irritable disposition (thought to be a problem of physical origin in Kampo medicine).

Consider This Formula If You Have Any of the Health Conditions Listed Above and Experience

Irritability, thirst for cold fizzy drinks, mouth sores, dark urine, and/or rapid pulse.

Energy Diagnosis

This formula is appropriate for an energy diagnosis of:

- Second Stage of Disease
- *Ki* deficiency

Gypsum and Atractylodis Formula

In the literature of modern Traditional Chinese Medicine this formula is usually called Maidservant from Yue Decoction Plus Atractylodis.

Japanese Name: Eppi-ka-jutsu-to
Chinese Name: Yue Bi Jia Zhu Tang
Scientific Name: Formula gypsum fibrosum et atractylodis lanceae

Common Brand Names

Atractylodis Combination (KPC Herbs, Lotus Classics, Qualiherb, Sun Ten)

Yue Bi Jia Zhu Tang (KPC Herbs, Lotus Classics, Qualiherb, Sun Ten)

Herbs Used to Make a Single Dose:

Gypsum 8.0 g
Ephedra Leaf 6.0 g
White Atractylodis Rhizome 4.0 g
Licorice Root 3.0 g
Jujube Fruit 2.0 g
Ginger (fresh) 1.0 g

Health Conditions Treated

Athralgia, arthritis, and eczema.

Who Should Use This Formula?

Physically active individuals who have arthritis or swollen joints.

Consider This Formula If You Have Any of the Health Conditions Listed Above and Experience

Joint pain, skin outbreaks, swelling, and / or scanty urination.

Energy Diagnosis

This formula is appropriate for an energy diagnosis of:

- *Ki* excess in the joints as disease makes the transition from first stage of Yang to second stage of Yang
- Stasis of fluids accumulated in joints

Comparisons to Other Formulas

Bupleurum and Magnolia Formula is more effective when there are Yang symptoms with tenderness on the right side of the abdomen.

Kudzu Formula offers more effective relief when there is stiff neck and back pain.

Stephania and Astragalus Formula is more effective when there are Yang symptoms, insufficient circulation of body fluids, loose stools, and thirst.

Hemp Seed Pill

Japanese Name: Mashinin-gan
Chinese Name: Ma Zi Ren Wan
Scientific Name: Formula cannabis

Common Brand Names

Apricot Seed & Linum Formula (KPC Herbs, Lotus Classics, Qualiherb, Sun Ten)
Ma Zi Ren Wan (KPC Herbs, Lotus Classics, Qualiherb, Sun Ten)

Herbs Used to Make a Single Dose

Rhubarb Root 4.0 g
Bitter Orange Fruit 2.0 g
Magnolia Bark 2.0 g
Peony Root 2.0 g
Marijuana Seed 5.0 g (Marijuana seed does not contain tetrahydrocannabonol, and will not cause a "high.")
Peach Seed 2.0 g

Health Conditions Treated

Constipation, especially in the elderly.

Who Should Use This Formula?

Relatively strong persons.

Consider This Formula If You Have Any of the Health Conditions Listed Above and Experience

Constipation with dry stool.

Energy Diagnosis

This formula is appropriate for an energy diagnosis of:

- Fourth Stage of Disease
- *Ki* neither deficient nor excessive

Honey-Fried Licorice Formula

Japanese Name: Shakanzo-to
Chinese Name: Zhi Gan Cao Tang
Scientific Name: Formula glycyrrhizae assusae

Common Brand Names

Baked Licorice Combination (Qualiherb)
Licorice (Baked) Combination (Sun Ten)
Licorice Combination (KPC Herbs, Lotus Classics)
Zhi Gan Cao Tang (KPC Herbs, Lotus Classics, Qualiherb, Sun Ten)

Herbs Used to Make a Single Dose

Rehmannia Root 6.0 g
Ophiopogon (Japanese Lily) Tuber 6.0 g
Cinnamon Bark 30
Jujube Fruit 3.0 g
Ginseng Root 3.0 g
Ginger (fresh) 1.0 g
Peony Root 3.0 g
Marijuana Seed 3.0 g (Marijuana seed does not contain tetrahydrocannabonol, and will not cause a "high.")
Gelatin 2.0 g

Health Conditions Treated

Asthma, chronic bronchitis, emphysema, and tachycardia (especially when caused by hyperthyroidism).

Who Should Use This Formula?

Persons whose physical activities are not yet limited by disease.

Consider This Formula If You Have Any of the Health Conditions Listed Above and Experience

Shortness of breath, extrasystole (extra heart beats), irregular pulse, fatigue, hot hands and feet, thirst, and/or tendency for constipation.

Energy Diagnosis

This formula is appropriate for an energy diagnosis of:

- Second Stage of Disease
- *Ki* deficiency causing distress in the chest

Japanese Lily Formula

Japanese Name: Bakumondo-to
Chinese Name: Mai Men Dong Tang
Scientific Name: Formula ophiopogonis

Common Brand Names

Mai Men Dong Tang (KPC Herbs, Lotus Classics, Qualiherb, Sun Ten)

Ophiopogon Combination (KPC Herbs, Lotus Classics, Qualiherb, Sun Ten)

Herbs Used to Make a Single Dose

Ophiopogon (Japanese Lily) Tuber 10.0 g
Pinellia Tuber 5.0 g
Jujube Fruit 5.0 g
Licorice Root 2.0 g
Ginseng 2.0 g
Rice 5.0 g

Health Conditions Treated

Bronchial asthma, bronchitis, and cough with sticky mucous secretion.

Who Should Use This Formula?

Persons of normal weight or greater with severe cough.

Consider This Formula If You Have Any of the Health Conditions Listed Above and Experience

Coughing spasms, red face, sticky phlegm, dry throat, shortness of breath, and/or lump in the throat. This formula is especially suitable for chronic cough during pregnancy and in the elderly.

Energy Diagnosis

This formula is appropriate for an energy diagnosis of:

- Second Stage of Disease
- Yang deficiency

Ligusticum Chuanxiong Powder to Be Taken with Green Tea

Japanese Name: Senkyu-chacho-san
Chinese Name: Chuan Xiong Cha Tiao San
Scientific Name: Pulvis theae et cnidii compositae

Common Brand Names

Cnidium & Tea Formula (KPC Herbs, Lotus Classics, Qualiherb, Sun Ten)

Chuan Xiong Cha Tiao San (KPC Herbs, Lotus Classics, Qualiherb, Sun Ten)

Herbs Used to Make a Single Dose

Ligusticum Root 3.0 g
Poria Mushroom 2.0 g
Mint Stem and Leaf 2.0 g
White Atractylodis Rhizome 2.0 g
Ledebouriella Root 2.0 g
Licorice Root 2.5 g
Notopterygium Rhizome 2.0 g
Green Tea 1.5 g

Chinese versions of this formula are meant to be taken with a cup of green tea. Japanese versions of this formula include the green tea in the formula.

Health Conditions Treated

Headache, lower back pain, migraine, and chronic sinusitis.

Who Should Use This Formula?

Relatively strong persons with conditions causing sharp pain.

Consider This Formula If You Have Any of the Health Conditions Listed Above and Experience

Headache, dizziness, blocked nose, joint and muscle pain, emotional instability, and/or painful tension of the back, neck, or shoulder muscles.

Energy Diagnosis

This formula is appropriate for an energy diagnosis of:

- First Stage of Disease
- *Ki* neither deficient nor excessive

Comparisons to Other Formulas

Cyperus and Perilla Powder may be more effective when there is nausea.

Ephedra, Asiasarum, and Prepared Aconite Formula may be more effective when there are chills and fatigue.

Minor Bluegreen Dragon Formula may be more effective when there is cough.

Major Order the Qi Formula

Japanese Name: Dai-joki-to
Chinese Name: Da Cheng Qi Tang
Scientific Name: Formula major ad auximillium vis vitalis

Common Brand Names

Da Cheng Qi Tang (KPC Herbs, Lotus Classics, Qualiherb, Sun Ten)

Major Rhubarb Combination (KPC Herbs, Lotus Classics, Qualiherb, Sun Ten)

Herbs Used to Make a Single Dose

Magnolia Bark 5.0 g
Bitter Orange (slices from whole fruit) 3.0 g
Rhubarb Root 2.0 g
Epsom Salts 1.5 g

Health Conditions Treated

Constipation, hypertension, and depression alternating with elation.

Who Should Use This Formula?

Physically active individuals.

Consider This Formula If You Have Any of the Health Conditions Listed Above and Experience

Bloating; gas; constipation with hard stools; thirst; restlessness, irritability, and/or excessive excitement with abdominal tension and a fast pulse.

Energy Diagnosis

This formula is appropriate for an energy diagnosis of:

- Third Stage of Disease
- Accumulation of heat

Minor Construct the Middle Decoction

Japanese Name: Sho-kenchu-to
Chinese Name: Xiao Jian Zhong Tang
Scientific Name: Formula salubritatis abdominis minor

Common Brand Names

Minor Cinnamon and Peony Combination (KPC Herbs, Lotus Classics, Qualiherb, Sun Ten)

Xiao Jian Zhong Tang (KPC Herbs, Lotus Classics, Qualiherb, Sun Ten)

Herbs Used to Make a Single Dose

Peony Root 6.0 g
Cinnamon Bark 4.0 g
Jujube Fruit 4.0 g
Licorice Root 2.0 g
Ginger (fresh) 2.0 g
Malt Sugar 20.0 g

Health Conditions Treated

Asthma, colic, excessive urination, chronic gastroenteritis, orthostatic hypotension (dizziness when moving from seated to standing position), and tonsillitis.

Who Should Use This Formula?

Children and adults who tire easily.

Consider This Formula If You Have Any of the Health Conditions Listed Above and Experience

Physical weakness, easy fatigue, abdominal pain, palpitations, nightsweats, nosebleeds, hot hands and feet, restlessness, and/or fearfulness.

Energy Diagnosis

This formula is appropriate for an energy diagnosis of:

- Fourth Stage of Disease
- Insufficient circulation of *ki* and blood in the digestive system causing spasms of the smooth muscle layers and the urinary tract

Comparisons to Other Formulas

Major Construct the Middle Formula may be more effective when muscle spasms are the primary symptom of concern.

Mysterious Decoction

Japanese Name: Shinpi-to
Chinese Name: Shen Mi Tang
Scientific Name: Formula divinitas

Common Brand Names

Ma Huang & Magnolia Combination (KPC Herbs, Lotus Classics, Qualiherb, Sun Ten)
Shen Mi Tang (KPC Herbs, Lotus Classics, Qualiherb, Sun Ten)

Herbs Used to Make a Single Dose

Ephedra Leaf 5.0 g
Peach Seed 4.0 g
Magnolia Bark 3.0 g
Bitter Orange Peel 2.5 g
Licorice Root 2.0 g
Bupleurum Root 2.0 g
Perilla Leaf 1.5 g

Health Conditions Treated

Asthma (especially children's asthma) bronchitis, colds, and emphysema.

Who Should Use This Formula?

Physically active individuals who have breathing difficulties.

Consider This Formula If You Have Any of the Health Conditions Listed Above and Experience

Cough, shortness of breath, moderate amounts of phlegm, moderate weakness of the digestive system, restlessness, nervousness, feeling of uprising heat, pain and moisture in the chest, and/or runny nose.

Energy Diagnosis

This formula is appropriate for an energy diagnosis of:

- Second Stage of Disease
- *Ki* congestion in the chest

Peach Pit Decoction to Order the Qi

Japanese Name: Tokaku-joki-to
Chinese Name: Tao He Cheng Qi Tang
Scientific Name: Formula persicae ad stimulationem vis vitalis

Common Brand Names

Persica & Rhubarb Combination (Qualiherb, Sun Ten)
Tao He Cheng Qi Tang (Qualiherb, Sun Ten)

Herbs Used to Make a Single Dose

Peach Seed 5.0 g
Cinnamon Bark 4.0 g
Rhubarb Root 3.0 g
Licorice Root 1.5 g
Epsom Salts 0.5 g

Health Conditions Treated

Endometriosis and pelvic inflammatory disease.

Who Should Use This Formula?

Women who have multiple physical complaints.

Consider This Formula If You Have Any of the Health Conditions Listed Above and Experience

Menstrual irregularities, constipation, hot flashes, hypertension, headache, painful tension of neck muscles with stiffness, and/or dizziness.

Energy Diagnosis

This formula is appropriate for an energy diagnosis of:

- Third Stage of Disease
- *Oketsu*

Comparisons to Other Formulas

Cinnamon and Poria Pill may be more effective when there are symptoms of emotional distress.

Goddess Powder may be more effective when fatigue and hot flashes are prominent symptoms.

Rhubarb and Moutan Formula may be more effective when there is gastritis.

Pinellia Draining Formula

This formula is also known as Pinellia Formula to Drain the Epigastrium. "Draining" refers to redirecting energies that have been misplaced upwards into the body.

Japanese Name: Hange-shashin-to
Chinese Name: Ban Xia Xie Xin Tang
Scientific Name: Formula pinelliae ad dispellandum et auxilium cordis

Common Brand Names

Ban Xia Xie Xin Tang (KPC Herbs, Qualiherb)
Pinellia Combination (KPC Herbs, Qualiherb)

Herbs Used to Make a Single Dose

Pinellia Tuber 5.0 g
Scutellaria Root 2.5 g
Licorice Root 2.5 g
Jujube Fruit 2.5 g
Ginseng Root 2.5 g
Coptis Rhizome 1.0 g
Ginger (dried) 2.5 g

Health Conditions Treated

Diarrhea, gastritis, nausea, vomiting, and mouth sores.

Who Should Use This Formula?

Physically active persons who experience digestive symptoms.

Consider This Formula If You Have Any of the Health Conditions Listed Above and Experience

Nausea, vomiting, loss of appetite, soft stool, occasional diarrhea, stress-induced stomach pain, loss of appetite, bloating, flatulence, and/or mild pain in the upper abdomen.

Energy Diagnosis

This formula is appropriate for an energy diagnosis of:

- Second Stage of Disease
- *Ki* neither deficient nor excessive

Comparisons to Other Formulas

Coptis Formula may be more effective when there is marked imbalance of *ki* distribution, such as red face and cold hands and feet.

Minor Construct the Middle Formula may be more effective when there is pain in the upper abdomen and/or "stomach rumbles."

Pinellia and Magnolia Bark Formula

Japanese Name: Hange-koboku-to
Chinese Name: Ban Xia Hou Po Tang
Scientific Name: Formula magnoliae et pinelliae

Common Brand Names

Ban Xia Hou Po Tang (Blue Light, Center for Natural Healing, Golden Flower Chinese Herbs, KPC Herbs, Qualiherb)
Pinellia & Magnolia (Kanpo, Qualiherb)
Pinellia & Magnolia Combination (Blue Light, Brion, Herbal Apothecary, KPC Herbs,
Ming Tong, Sheng Chang)
Pinellia & Magnolia Bark (Golden Flower Chinese Herbs)

Herbs Used to Make a Single Dose

Pinellia Tuber 6.0 g
Poria Mushroom 5.0 g
Magnolia Bark 3.0 g
Perilla Leaf 2.0 g
Ginger (fresh) 1.0 g

Health Conditions Treated

Gastritis, hoarseness, and laryngitis (especially when triggered by emotional stress).

Who Should Use This Formula?

Women in the first trimester of pregnancy, physically active persons with good color.

Consider This Formula If You Have Any of the Health Conditions Listed Above and Experience

Hoarseness, lump in the throat, insomnia, palpitations, shortness of breath, cough, and/or the sound of fluctuating liquid in the stomach or above the stomach.

Energy Diagnosis

This formula is appropriate for an energy diagnosis of:

- Second Stage of disease
- *Ki* neither excessive nor deficient; localized deficiency of *ki* in the throat causing lump in the throat.

Platycodon Formula

Japanese Name: Kikkyo-to
Chinese Name: Jie Geng Wan
Scientific Name: Formula platycodi

Common Brand Names

Jie Geng Wan (Asian Patents)
Jie Geng Tang (Lotus Classics)
Platycodon Formula (Lotus Classics)
Platycodon Pill (Asian Patents)

Herbs Used to Make a Single Dose

Licorice Root 3.0 g
Platycodon 2.0 g

Health Conditions Treated

Laryngitis, sore throat, and tonsillitis.

Who Should Use This Formula?

Since both of the herbs in this formula are of neutral energy, the formula is suitable for anyone suffering sore throat.

Consider This Formula If You Have Any of the Health Conditions Listed Above and Experience

Hoarseness, sore throat, lump in the throat, difficulty swallowing, phlegm, and/or inflamed tonsils.

Energy Diagnosis

This formula is appropriate for an energy diagnosis of:

- Second Stage of Disease
- *Ki* neither deficient nor excessive

Comparisons to Other Formulas

Kudzu Formula should be added if there is tension in the muscles of the shoulders or neck.

Regulate the Stomach and Order the Qi Formula

Japanese Name: Choi-joki-to
Chinese Name: Tiao Wei Cheng Qi Tang
Scientific Name: Formula animationis stomachi

Common Brand Names

Rhubarb & Mirabilitum (KPC Herbs, Qualiherb)
Tiao Wei Cheng Qi Tang (KPC Herbs, Qualiherb)

Herbs Used to Make a Single Dose

Rhubarb Root 2.0 g
Licorice Root 1.5 g
Epsom Salts 0.5 g

Health Conditions Treated

Constipation.

Who Should Use This Formula?

Relatively strong persons for whom constipation is the only health complaint.

Consider This Formula If You Have Any of the Health Conditions Listed Above and Experience

Constipation, bloating, thirst, and/or tendency for fever.

Energy Diagnosis

This formula is appropriate for an energy diagnosis of:

- Third Stage of Disease
- *Ki* excess in the intestine

Comparisons to Other Formulas

Hemp Seed Pill may be more effective if stools are soft but the muscles of the lower digestive tract are too weak to allow them to be passed.

Restore the Spleen Formula

"Restoring the spleen" refers to reinvigorating the energies of the digestive tract.

Japanese Name: Kihi-to
Chinese Name: Gui Pi Tang
Latin Name: Formula lienalis angelicae

Common Brand Names

Gather Vitality (Kan Herbals)
Ginseng & Longan (Qualiherb)
Ginseng & Longan Combination (KPC Herbs, Lotus Classics, Sun Ten)
Ginseng & Longan Formula (Chinese Classics, Golden Flower Chinese Herbs)
Gui Pi Tang (Chinese Classics, Golden Flower Chinese Herbs, Health Concerns, Kan Herbals, KPC Herbs, Lotus Classics, Qualiherb, Sun Ten)
Shen Gem (Health Concerns)

Herbs Used to Make a Single Dose

Astragalus Root 3.0 g
Ginseng Root 3.0 g
White Atractylodis Root 3.0 g
Poria Mushroom 3.0 g
Longan Fruit 2.0 g
Jujube Fruit 2.0 g
Dong Quai Root 2.0 g
Licorice Root 1.0 g

Ginger (fresh) 1.0 g
Aucklandia Root 1.0 g
Gardenia Fruit 3.0 g
Polygala Root 3.0 g

Health Conditions Treated

Depression, stress-induced heartburn, insomnia, memory problems, and recurrent nosebleed.

Who Should Use This Formula?

Physically weak persons whose daily routine is interrupted by illness.

Consider This Formula If You Have Any of the Health Conditions Listed Above and Experience

Racing heart, palpitations, forgetfulness, insomnia, sometimes bloody stool, night sweats, loss of appetite, and/or "jelly belly" (markedly reduced abdominal tension).

Energy Diagnosis

This formula is appropriate for an energy diagnosis of:

- Fourth Stage of Disease
- *Ki* deficiency

Comparisons to Other Formulas

Augmented Restore the Spleen Formula is more effective when primary symptoms of concern are mood swings, irritability, and/or feeling of uprising heat.Ten-Significant Tonic Formula is more effective when there is marked coldness throughout the body; may be most effective when psychic symptoms are not yet evident.

Warming and Clearing Formula is more effective when psychic symptoms are severe and there is redness in the face and/or a tendency to fever.

Rhubarb and Licorice Formula

Japanese Name: Daio-kanzo-to
Chinese Name: Da Huang Gan Cao Tang
Scientific Name: Formula glycyrrhizae et rhei

Common Brand Names

Da Huang Gan Cao Tang (Brion)
Daio-kanzo-to (Honso,* Tsumura)
Kampo4Digestive Smooth Laxative (Honso*)
(*Made in Japan)

Herbs Used to Make a Single Dose

Rhubarb Root 4.0 g
Licorice Root 2.0 g

Health Conditions Treated

Constipation, and also traveller's diarrhea.

Who Should Use This Formula?

Physically active individuals prone to constipation.

Consider This Formula If You Have Any of the Health Conditions Listed Above and Experience

Constipation without other symptoms, or suspected exposure to spoiled food or contaminated water.

Energy Diagnosis

This formula is appropriate for an energy diagnosis of:

- First Stage of Disease
- *Ki* deficiency localized in the intestines

Rhubarb and Moutan Formula

Japanese Name: Daio-botanpi-to
Chinese Name: Da Huang Mu Dan Tang
Latin Name: Formula moutan et rhei

Common Brand Names

Da Huang Mu Dan Tang (KPC Herbs, Lotus Classics, Qualiherb)
Rhubarb & Moutan (Qualiherb)
Rhubarb & Moutan Combination (KPC Herbs, Lotus Classics)

Herbs Used to Make a Single Dose

Peach Seed 4.0 g
Moutan Root 4.0 g
Rhubarb Root 2.0 g
Benincasa Seed 6.0 g
Epsom Salts 1.8

Health Conditions Treated

Crohn's disease, constipation, dysmenorrhea, heavy periods, and hemorrhoids.

Who Should Use This Formula?

Relatively strong persons who experience distention of the abdomen with other symptoms.

Consider This Formula If You Have Any of the Health Conditions Listed Above and Experience

Constipation, abdominal distention, inflammation of the pelvic region, and/or inflammation of the intestines.

Energy Diagnosis

This formula is appropriate for an energy diagnosis of:

- Third Stage of Disease
- Localized *ki* stasis

Comparisons to Other Formulas

Cinnamon and Poria Pill may be more effective when there is heat in the upper part of the body and cold in the lower part of the body, or after constipation has been corrected but other symptoms remain.

Six-Gentlemen Formula

Japanese Name: Rikkunshi-to
Chinese Name: Liu Jun Zi Tang
Scientific Name: Formula medicamentorum sextoum nobilis

Common Brand Names

Liu Jun Zi Tang (KPC Herbs, Qualiherb)
Six Major Herb Formula (KPC Herbs, Qualiherb)

Herbs Used to Make a Single Dose

Ginseng Root 4.0 g
Pinellia Tuber 4.0 g
Poria Mushroom 4.0 g
Jujube Fruit 2.0 g
Bitter Orange Peel 2.0 g
White Atractylodis Root 2.0 g
Licorice Root 1.0 g
Ginger (fresh) 0.5 g

Health Conditions Treated

Chronic gastritis, irritable bowel syndrome, and peptic ulcer.

Who Should Use This Formula?

Physically inactive persons who experience digestive problems.

Consider This Formula If You Have Any of the Health Conditions Listed Above and Experience

Loss of appetite, bloating, abdominal distention, cold hands and feet, fatigue, and/or "stomach rumbles."

Energy Diagnosis

This formula is appropriate for an energy diagnosis of:

- Fourth Stage of Disease
- *Ki* deficiency

Comparisons to Other Formulas

The overuse of this formula may result in a dry mouth, thirst, and irritability. It should not be used when there is fever. Alternative formulas include:

- Four-Gentlemen Formula, when there are no "stomach rumbles."
- Ginseng Formula, when there is diarrhea with runny stools, cold arms and legs.
- Tonify the Middle and Augment the Qi Formula, when there is mild fever.

Two-Cured Formula

Japanese Name: Nichin-to
Chinese Name: Er Chen Tang
Scientific Name: Formula aurantii nobilis percarpium

Common Brand Names

Citrus & Pinellia Combination (KPC Herbs, Lotus Classics)

Citrus & Pinellia Formula (Chinese Classics, Golden Flower Chinese Herbs)

Er Chen Tang (Chinese Classics, Golden Flower Chinese Herbs, KPC Herbs, Lotus Classics, Qualiherb, Sun Ten, Three Treasures)

Limpid Sea (Three Treasures)

Herbs Used to Make a Single Dose

Pinellia Tuber 5.0 g
Poria Mushroom 5.0 g
Chen-pi Peel 4.0 g
Licorice Root 1.0 g
Ginger (fresh) 1.0 g

Health Conditions Treated

Acute and chronic gastritis and morning sickness.

Who Should Use This Formula?

Persons with tendency for obesity.

Consider This Formula If You Have Any of the Health Conditions Listed Above and Experience

Nausea, gastric pain, dizziness, racing pulse, headache, and/or rumbling stomach.

Energy Diagnosis

This formula is appropriate for an energy diagnosis of:

- Fourth Stage of Disease
- *Ki* deficiency
- Yin excess

Comparisons to Other Formulas

Six-Gentlemen Formula may be more effective if nausea is the predominant symptom.

Warm the Menses Formula

("Warming the menses" refers to supplying the uterus with enough energy that blood flows in its normal channels, rather than leaking downward.)

Japanese Name: Unkei-to
Chinese Name: Wen Jing Tang
Scientific Name: Formula orbis tepefactum

Common Brand Names

Dang Gui & Evodia (Qualiherb)
Tangkuei & Evodia Combination (KPC Herbs, Lotus Classics, Sun Ten)
Warm the Menses (Women's Treasure)
Wen Jing Tang (KPC Herbs, Lotus Classics, Qualiherb, Sun Ten, Women's Treasure)

Herbs Used to Make a Single Dose

Ophiopogon (Japanese Lily) Tuber 4.0 g

Pinellia Tuber 4.0 g
Dong Quai Root 3.0 g
Licorice Root 2.0 g
Cinnamon Bark 2.0 g
Peony Root 2.0 g
Ligusticum Root 2.0 g
Ginseng Root 2.0 g
Moutan Root 2.0 g
Evodia Fruit 1.0 g
Ginger (fresh) 1.0 g
Gelatin 2.0 g

Health Conditions Treated

Amenorrhea, dysmenorrhea, menopausal discomforts (especially hot flashes), and eczema.

Who Should Use This Formula?

Women who exhibit Yin characteristics, such as pale complexion, chronic fatigue, soft muscles, etc.

Consider This Formula If You Have Any of the Health Conditions Listed Above and Experience

Bleeding between menstrual periods or no periods at all, hot flashes, hot hands, dry lips and skin, coldness in lower abdomen, loss of tone in abdominal muscles, bloating, abdominal pain, and/or diarrhea due to *oketsu* syndrome. While most of the body exhibits Yin, there may be localized excesses of Yang causing dry lips and skin, hot hands and feet, red face, and hot flashes.

Energy Diagnosis

This formula is appropriate for an energy diagnosis of:

- Second Stage of Disease
- *Ki* deficiency

Warming and Clearing Formula

Japanese Name: Unsei-in
Chinese Name: Wen Qing Yin
Scientific Name: Decoctum dispelentis tepefactum

Common Brand Names

Dang Gui & Gardenia (Qualiherb)
Tang-kuei & Gardenia (Lotus Classics)
Tangkuei & Gardenia Combination (KPC Herbs, Sun Ten)
Wen Qing Yin (KPC Herbs, Lotus Classics, Qualiherb, Sun Ten)

Herbs Used to Make a Single Dose

Rehmannia Root 3.0 g
Peony Root 3.0 g
Ligusticum Root 3.0 g
Dong Quai Root 3.0 g
Scutellaria Root 1.5 g
Phellodendron Bark 1.5 g
Coptis Rhizome 1.5 g
Gardenia Fruit 1.5 g

Health Conditions Treated

Eczema, dermatitis, psoriasis, bleeding hemorrhoids, hives, canker sores, and hot flashes.

Who Should Use This Formula?

Persons whose daily activities are not limited by any health conditions.

Consider This Formula If You Have Any of the Health Conditions Listed Above and Experience

Dry skin; hives or rashes; freckles; feeling of uprising heat; hot hands and feet; emotional hypersensitivity; tendency to hemorrhage anywhere in the body (nosebleed, bleeding between periods, or bleeding hemorrhoids); red skin, reduced glandular activity; and/or itch.

Energy Diagnosis

This formula is appropriate for an energy diagnosis of:

- Second Stage of Disease
- *Ki* neither excessive nor deficient
- *Oketsu*

Comparisons to Other Formulas

Coptis Antidote may be more effective if sensation of heat is the most prominent symptom.

White Tiger Formula

Japanese Name: Byakko-to
Chinese Name: Bai Hu Tang
Scientific Name: Formula tigridis albi

Common Brand Names

Bai Hu Tang (KPC Herbs, Lotus Classics, Qualiherb, Sun Ten)
Byakko-to (Honso,* Tsumura*)
Gypsum Combination (KPC Herbs, Lotus Classics, Qualiherb, Sun Ten)
(*Made in Japan)

Herbs Used to Make a Single Dose

Gypsum 15.0 g
Anemarrhena Root 5.0 g
Licorice Root 2.0 g
Sticky Rice 8.0 g

Health Conditions Treated

Gum disease (periodontitis).

Who Should Use This Formula?

Physically active individuals experiencing acute symptoms of the health conditions listed above.

Consider This Formula If You Have Any of the Health Conditions Listed Above and Experience

Feeling of heat in the entire body, fever, thirst, sweating, and/or skin eruptions.

Energy Diagnosis

This formula is appropriate for an energy diagnosis of:

- Third Stage of Disease
- Yang symptoms
- *Ki* excess

Comparisons to Other Formulas

Five-Ingredient Powder with Poria may be taken with this formula when there is diarrhea, nausea, or vomiting.

Polyporus Formula may be more effective when there is scanty urination.

Tonify the Middle and Augument the *Qi* Formula may be a helpful addition when there are also kidney problems.

Glossary

BLOOD. A broad term to describe the physical blood in the body that moistens the muscles, tissues, skin and hair, as well as nourishing the cells and organs

BLOOD DEFICIENCY. A lack of blood with signs of anemia, dizziness, dry skin or hair, scant or absent menstruation, fatigue, pale skin and poor memory

CHANNELS. The twelve major pathways through which *ki* flows, supplying energy and nourishment to the body

COLD. Decreased function of an organ system or of the body as a whole; in Japan, feeling run down.

DAMP HEAT. Condition of dampness and heat combined, causing

thick yellow secretions and phlegm, or yellow coloration (jaundice) or inflammation of the skin

DAMPNESS. Excessive fluids in a tissue or organ system, manifesting itself as abdominal bloating, loss of appetite, nausea, vomiting, feeling heavy or sluggish, and stiff, aching or sore joints

DECOCTION. A combination of herbs prepared in boiling water

DEFICIENCY. Insufficiency of *ki*, blood, Yang, or Yin

EXCESS. Too much heat, cold, damp, Yang, or Yin

EXTERNAL. Location of illnesses such as fevers and skin eruptions/on the surface of the body

FIRE. Energy disturbance resulting from overactivity of the internal organs or from extreme emotion, typically causing fever, red or bloodshot eyes, swelling, sore throat and flushed face

FIVE ELEMENTS. The five energies of wood, earth, metal, water and fire

HEART. Energy organ responsible for blood circulation

INTERNAL. Location of illnesses such as those that affect *ki*, blood, and organs inside the body

KI. Pronounced "kee," the vital energy or life force that flows through the meridians and is used to protect, transform, and warm the body

KI DEFICIENCY. Lack of *ki* which is seen with symptoms of lethargy, weakness, shortness of breath, slow metabolism, frequent colds and flu with slow recovery, low or soft voice, palpitations, and/or frequent urination

KIDNEY. Energy organ encompassing urinary and reproductive systems, growth and development, endocrine system, hormones, brain and nervous system, metabolism, bones, hair, and respiratory functions

LIVER. Energy organ regulating storage of blood and creating harmony in mental and emotional states

LUNG. Energy organ in charge of respiration, water metabolism, blood circulation and some functions of the immune system

ORGANS. Grouping of energies roughly associated with an anatomical organ

PHLEGM. Either a visible, sticky substance such as mucus or a localized energy disturbance that causes a reduction in the flow of *ki*

SEVEN EMOTIONS. Sadness, fright, fear, grief, anger, joy (extreme excitability), and pensiveness, regarded as potential causes of illness

SIX EXTERNAL EVILS. Include wind, cold, summerheat, dampness, dryness, and fire, regarded as potential causes of illness

SPLEEN. Energy organ responsible for transformation of food and water

STASIS. A blockage or buildup of *ki* or blood that prevents it from flowing freely, a precursor of disease

SUMMERHEAT. Overexertion of an organ system resulting in symptoms of thirst, aversion to heat and craving for cold, infection, inflammation, dryness, red face, sweating, irritability, dark yellow urine, and nervous tension

TCM. Abbreviation for Traditional Chinese Medicine

TONIFY. To nourish, support or strengthen the condition of life, blood or weak organ function

TOXICITY. Applies to any inflammation, infection or severe heat disease, or energy residue of anger, fear, or "burning" emotion

WEI QI. Defensive energy, the TCM equivalent of the immune system

WIND. Causes the sudden movement of a condition

YANG. Represents heat and the body's ability to generate and maintain warmth and circulation

YANG DEFICIENCY. A cold condition due to lack of the heating quality of yang, manifesting itself as lethargy, poor digestion, cold, lower back pain and decreased sex drive

YANG SYMPTOMS. Rapid pulse, hypertension, aggressive actions, loud voice, high fever, red complexion or restlessness

YIN. Represents cool and the substance of the body, including blood and bodily fluids that nurture and moisten the organs and tissues

YIN DEFICIENCY. A heat condition that results in symptoms of night sweats, fever, nervous exhaustion, dry eyes and throat, dizziness, blurred vision, insomnia and a burning sensation in the palms of the hands, soles of the feet, and the chest

YIN SYMPTOMS. Excessive fluids in the body causing fluid retention, a plump or swollen appearance, or lethargy

References

Aconite

1. Ikeda, Y., Oyama, T., Taki, M., "Effect of processed Aconiti tuber on catecholamine and indoleamine contents in brain in rats," *Acta Anaesthesiologica Belgica*, 45(3), 113-118 (1994).
2. Tang, X. C., Zhu, M. Y., Feng, J., Wang, Y. E., "Studies on pharmacologic effects of lappaconitine hydrobromide," *Acta Pharmacologica Sinica*, 18, 579-584 (1983).
3. Oyama, T., Isono, T., Suzuki, Y., Hayakawa, Y., "Anti-nociceptive effects of aconiti tuber and its alkaloids," *American Journal of Chinese Medicine*, 22(2), 175-182 (1994).

Angelica Formula

1. Yanase, T., Nishizawa, K., Inoue, O., Sukamoto, T., Saito, Y., "Antinociceptive effects of *Kami-kihi-to in mice*," (in Japanese, available as abstract on MedLine) *Nippon Yakurigaku Zasshi*, 108(2), 77-83 (August 1996).
2. Yamaguchi, K., Kido, H., Kawakatsu, T., Fukuroi, T., Suzuki, M., Yanabu, M., Nomura. S., Kokawa, T., Yasunaga, K., "Effects of *kami-kihi-to* (jia-wei-gui-pi-tang) on autoantibodies in patients with chronic immune thrombocytopenic purpura," *American Journal of Chinese Medicine*, 21(3-4), 251-255 (1993).

Artemisia and Poria Five-Ingredient Powder

1. Chen Z., "Clinical study of 96 cases with chronic hepatitis B treated with jiedu yanggan gao by a double-blind method" (in Chinese, available as abstract on Medline), *Zhong Xi Yi Jie He Za Zhi*, 10(2), 71-74 (February 1990).

2. Tokoro, T., "Developmental mechanism of low myopia and therapeutic possibilities. A review" (in Japanese, available as abstract on Medline), *Nippon Ganka Gakkai Zasshi*, 102(12), 796-812 (December 1998).

Astragalus Formula

1. Chen, L.X., Liao, J.Z., Guo, W.Q., "Effects of *Astragalus membranaceus* on left ventricular function and oxygen free radical in acute myocardial infarction patients and mechanism of its cardiotonic action," *Chung-Kuo Chung Hsi I Chieh Ho Tsa Chih—Chinese Journal of Modern Developments in Traditional Medicine*, 15(3), 141-143 (March 1995).
2. Huang, W.M., Yan, J., Xu, J., "Clinical and experimental study on inhibitory effect of sanhuang mixture on platelet aggregation," *Chung-Kuo Chung Hsi I Chieh Ho Tsa Chih—Chinese Journal of Modern Developments in Traditional Medicine*, 15(8), 465-467 (August 1995).
3. Shi, H.M., Dai, R.H., Fan, W.H., "Intervention of lidocaine and *Astragalus membranaceus* on ventricular late potentials," *Chung-Kuo Chung Hsi I Chieh Ho Tsa Chih—Chinese Journal of Modern Developments in Traditional Medicine*, 14(10), 598-600 (October 1994).
4. Nagano, T., Itoh, H., Takeyama, M., "Effect of *Dai-kenchu-to* on levels of 3 brain-gut peptides (motilin, gastrin and somatostain) in human plasma," *Biological Pharmacology Bulletin*, 22(10), 1131-1133 (October 1999).
5. Satoh, K., Kase, Y., Hayakawa, T., Murata, P., Ishige, A., Sasaki, H., "*Dai-kenchu-to* accelerates small intestine movement," *Biological Pharmacology Bulletin*, 24(10), 1122-1126 (October 2001).
6. Hayakawa, T., Kase, Y., Saito, K., Hashimoto, K., Ishige, A., Komatsu, Y., Sasaki, H., "Effects of *Dai-kenchu-to* on intestinal obstruction following laparotomy," *Journal of Smooth Muscle Research*, 35(2), 47-54 (April 1999).
7. Yan, M., Song, H., Xie, N., Zhang, L., "Changes of intestinal flora in senile mouse models and the antagonistic activity of the root of *Astragalus membraceus* (Fisch) Bge.," *Chung Kuo Chung Yao Tsa Chih*, 20(10), 624-626, inside backcover (October 1995).
8. Chen, Y.C., "Experimental studies on the effects of *danggui buxue* decoction of IL-2 production of blood-deficient mice," *Chung Kuo Chung Yao Tsa Chih*, 19(12), 739-741, 763 (December 1994).

Augmented Rambling Powder

1. Tanaka, T., "Effects of herbal medicines on menopausal symptoms induced by gonadtropin-releasing hormone agonist therapy," *Clinical and Experimental Obstetrics and Gynecology*, 28(1), 20-23 (2001).
2. Ishikawa, T., Funahashi, T., Kudo, J., "Effectiveness of the Kampo *kami-shoyo-san* (TJ-24) for tremor of antipsychotic-induced parkinsonism," *Psychiatry and Clinical Neuroscience*, 54(5), 579-582 (October 2000).

Bupleurum and Magnolia Formula

1. Koda, A., Nishiyori, T. Nagai, H., Matsuura, N., Tsuchiya, H., "Anti-allergic actions of traditional Oriental medicine-actions against types I and IV hypersensitivity reactions," *Nippon Yakurigaku Zasshi*, 80(1), 31-41 (July 1982).
2. Kobayashi, S., et al, "Bronchia asthma and the efficacy of *saiboku-to*," *Wakan-Yaku Zasshi*, 2, 598 (1985).
3. Egashira, Y., et al, "On the action of *saiboku-to* in patients suffering from bronchial asthma long-time treatment and effect on the adreno-cortico-pituitary system," *Wakan-Yaku Zasshi*, 2, 158 (1985).
4. Nakajima, S., Tohda, Y., Ohkawa, K., Chihara, J., Nagasaka, Y., "Effect of *saiboku-to* (TJ-96) on bronchial asthma. Induction of glucocorticoid receptor, beta-adrenaline receptor, IgE-Fc epsilon receptor expression and its effect on experimental immediate and late asthmatic reaction." *Annals of the New York Academy of Sciences*, 685, 549-560 (23 June 1993).
5. Homma, M., Oka, K., Kobayashi, H., Niitsuma, T., Yamamoto, S., Itoh, H., Takahashi, N., "Impact of free magnolol excretions in asthmatic patients who responded well to *saiboku-to*, a Chinese herbal medicine," *Japanese Journal of Pharmacology*, 45(9), 844-846 (September 1993).
6. Yuzuribara, M., Ikarashi, Y., Ishihara, K., Kushida, H., Ishige, A., Sasaki, H., Maruyama, Y., "Effects of subacutely administered *saiboku-to*, an Oriental herbal medicine, on pharamcodynamics and pharmcokinetics of diazepam in rodents," *European Journal of Drug Metabolism and Pharmacokinetics*, 25(2), 127-136 (April-June 2000).
7. Maruyama, Y., Kuribara, H, Morita, M, Mitsutoshi, Y., Weintraub, S. T., "Identification of Magnolol and Honokiol as Anxiolytic Agents in Extracts of *Saiboku-to*, an Oriental herbal Medicine," *Journal of Natural Products*, 61, 135-138 (1998).

Bupleurum and Poria Formula

1. Ikeda, K., Takasaka, T., "Treatment of secretory otitis media with kampo medicine," *Archives of Otorhinolaryngology*, 245(4), 234-236 (1988).
2. O-Uchi, T., Kanzaki, J., Tsuchihashi, N., "Clinical analysis of steroid-responsive sensorineural hearing loss," *Auris Nasus Larynx*, 20(2), 79-93 (1993).
3. Borigini, M., et al, "TJ-114 (Sairei-to), an herbal Medicine in Rheumatoid Arthritis: A Preliminary 'Go-No Go' Clinical Trial," *Journal of Clinical Rheumatology*, 2, 203 (December 1996).
4. Nakayama, S., Matsushita, A., Ichiba, S., Yabe, H., Nagai, K., "Clinical evaluation of traditional Chinese medicine for chronic idiopathic thrombocytopenic purpura," *Rinsho Kesueki*, 33(2), 157-161 (February 1992).
5. Motoo, Y., Taga, H., Yamaguichi, Y., Wtanabe, H., Okai, T., Sawabu, N., "Effect of *niuche-she-qi-wan* on painful muscle cramps in patients with liver cirrhosis: a preliminary report," *American Journal of Chinese Medicine*, 25(1), 97-102 (1997).

6. Tozawa, K., Akita, H., Yamamoto, H., Nakahira, Y., Kawai, T., Kohei, K., "Clinical efficacy of *sairei-to* in preventionof recurrence of urethral stenosis: report of two cases," *Hinyokika Kiyo*, 44(1), 49-51 (January 1998).
7. Yoshikawa, N., Ito, H., Takekoshi, Y., Honda, M., Awazu, M., Iijima, K., Nakamura, H., Seio, K., Takeda, N., Hattori, S., Matsuda, I., "Standard versus long-term prednisolone with *sairei-to* for initial therapy in childhood steroid-responsive nephrotic syndrome: a prospective controlled study," *Nippon Jinzo Gakkai Shi*, 40(8), 587-590 (November 1998).

Bupleurum Formula to Purify the Liver

1. Sasaki, T., Ohta, S., Kamogawa, A., Shinoda, M., "Protective effects of various Chinese traditional medicines against experimental cholestasis," *Chemical Pharmacology Bulletin*, 38(2), 513-516 (February 1990).
2. Yamasaki, K., Kajimura, K., Nakano, M., Yokoyama, H., Yoneda, K., Umezawa, C., "Effects of preparations of Chinese medicinal prescriptions on digestive enzymes in vitro and in vivo," *Biological Pharmacology Bulletin*, 21(2), 133-139 (February 1998).
3. Hiai, S., Yokoyama, H., Nagasawa, T., Oura, H., "Stimulation of the pituitary-adrenocortical axis by saikosaponin of Bupleuri radix," *Chemical Pharmaceutical Bulletin*, 29, 495-499 (1981).
4. Inoue, T., Suigimoto, Y., Masuda, H., Kamei, C., "Antiallergic effect of flavonoid glycosides obtained from *Mentha piperita L.*," *Biological Pharmacology Bulletin*, 25(2), 256–259 (February 2002).
5. Wang, Y.C., Brian, R.L., Zhou, H.L., "Effects of neutrophils on histamine release from mast cells," *Zhongguo Yao Li Xue Bao*, 11(3), 285–288 (May 1990).

Cinnamon Formula

1. Cohen, S., Tyrrell, D.A., Smith, A.P., "Psychological stress and susceptibility to the common cold," *New England Journal of Medicine*. 325(9), 606-612 (29 August 1991).
2. Singh, H. B., Srivastava, M., Singh , A. B., Srivastava, A. K.., "Cinnamon bark oil, a potent fungitoxicant against fungi causing respiratory tract mycoses," *Allergy*, 50(12), 995-999 (December 1995).
3. Huang, K. C. *The Pharmacology of Chinese Herbs* (Boca Raton, Florida: CRC Press, 1993), p. 209.
4. Yamahara, J., Hatakeyama, S., Taniguchi, K., Kawamura, M., "Stomachic principles in ginger. II. Pungent and anti-effects of low polar constituents isolated from ginger, dried rhizome of *Zingiber officinale* Roscoe cultivated in Taiwan. The absolute stereostructure of a new diarylheptanoid," *Yakugaku Zasshi—Journal of the Pharmaceutical Society of Japan*, 112(9), 645-655 (September 1992).
5. Yao, G. S., Li, Y. J., Chang, X. Q., Lu, J. H., "Vitamin C content in vegetables and fruits in the Shenyang (China) market during four seasons," *Acta Nutritica Sinica*, 5, 373-379 (1983).
6. Bensky, D., Gamble, A., Bensky, L., Kaptchuk, T. *Chinese Herbal Medicine: Materia Medica, Revised Edition* (Seattle: Eastland Press, 1992), p. 323.

7. Chen, M. F., et. al., "Effect of glycyrrhizin on the pharmacokinetics of prednisolone following low dosage of prednisolone hemisuccinate," *Endocronologica Japonica*, 37, 331-341 (1990).
8. Xu, F.H., Uebaba, K., Cyong, C.Y., "Effects of Kampo formulations (Chinese herbal medicine traditionally used in Japan) on event-related electric potentials," *Acupuncture and Electrotherapy Research*, 24(2), 89-104 (1999).

Clear Summerheat and Augment the Qi Formula

1. Hagino, K., Oshige, H., Ozawa, K., Kudo, K., Koide, M., Sugita, R., Adachi, K., Koike, H., "Effect of XKJ-001, a crude drug preparation, on body water distribution and water excretion in mice," *Yakugaku Zasshi*, 111(6), 293-298 (June 1991).

Coptis Antidote

1. Takase, H., Miura, Ok, Ito, K., "Pharmacological studies of some blended traditional Chinese medicines on gastric functions. (1). The effects of oren-gedoku-to (OGT), san'o-syasin-to (SST), antyu-san (AS) and dai-saiko-to (DS) on ethanol- and aspirin-induced injury of gastric mucosal barrier," *Nippon Yakurigaku Zasshi*, 89(5), 299-306 (1991).
2. Mori, M., Hojo, E., Takano, K., "Action of *oren-gedoku-to* on platelet aggregation in vitro," *American Journal of Chinese Medicine*, 19(2), 131-143 (1991).
3. Fushitani, S., Minakuchi, K., Tsuchiya, K., Takasugi, M., Murakami, K., "Studies on attenuation of post-ischemic brain injury by kampo medicines—inhibitory effects of free radical production," *Yakugaku Zasshi*, 115(8), 611-617 (August 1995).
4. Yotsumoto, H., Yanagita, T., Yamamoto, K., Ogawa, Y., Cha, J.Y., Mori, Y., "Inhibitory effects of *oren-gedoku-to* and its components on cholesteryl ester synthesis in cultured human hepatocyte HepG2 cells: evidence from the cultured HepG2 cells and in vitro assay of ACAT," *Planta Medica*, 63(2), 141-145 (April 1997).
5. Miura, N., Yamamoto, M., Ueki, T., Kitani, T., Fukuda, K, Komatsu, Y., "Inhibition of thymocyte apoptosis by berberine," *Biochemical Pharmacology*, 53(9), 1315-1322 (May 1997).
6. Kondo, Y., Kondo, F., Asanuma, M., Tanaka, K., Ogawa, N., "Protective effect of *oren-gedoku-to* against induction of neuronal death by transient cerebral ischemia in the C57BL/6 mouse," *Neurochemical Research*, 25(2), 205-209 (February 2000).
7. Fukutake, M., Miura, N., Yamamoto, M., Fukuda, K., Iijima, O., Ishikawa, H., Kubo, M., Okada, M., Komastsu, Y., Sasaki, H., Wakabayashi, K., Ishige, A., Amagaya, S., "Suppressive effect of the herbal medicine *Oren-gedoku-to* on cyclooxygenase-2 activity and azoxymethane-induced aberrant crypt foci development in rats," *Cancer Letters*, 157(1), 9-14 (August 2000).
8. Nose, M., Sakushima, J., Harada, D., Ogihara, Y., "Comparison of immunopharmacological actions of 8 kinds of kampo-hozais clinically used in atopic dermatitis on delayed-type hypersensitivity in mice," *Biological Pharmacology Bulletin*, 22(1), 48-54 (January 1999).

9. Zhou, H., Mineshita, S., "The effect of *oren-gedoku-to* on experimental colitis in rats," *Japanese Journal of Pharmacology*, 51(9), 1065-1074 (September 1999).
10. Xu, J., Murakami, Y., Matsumoto, K., Tohda, M., Watanabe, H., Zhang, S., Yu, Q., Shen, J., "Protective effect of *Oren-gedoku*-to (Huang-Lian-Jie-Du-Tang) against impairment of learning and memory induced by transient cerebral ischemia in mice," *Journal of Ethnopharmacology*, 73(3) 405-413 (December 2000).

Dong Quai and Gentian Formula

1. Yamasaki, K., Kajimura, K., Nakano, M., Yokoyama, H., Yoneda, K., Umezawa, C., "Effects of preparations of Chinese medicinal prescriptions on digestive enzymes in vitro and in vivo," *Biological Pharmacology Bulletin*, 21(2) 133-139 (February 1998).

Dong Quai and Peony Formula

1. Usuki, S., "Effects of *hachimijiogan*, *tokishakuyakusan*, *keishibukuryogan*, *ninjinto* and *unkeito* on estrogen and progesterone secretion in preovulatory follicles incubated in vitro," *American Journal of Chinese Medicine*, 19(1), 65-71 (1991).
2. Irahara, M., Yasui, T., Tezuka, M., Ushigoe, K., Yamano, S., Kamada, M., Anono, T., "Evidence that Toki-shakuyaku-san and its ingedients enhance the secretion of a cytokine-induced neutrophil chemoattractant (CINC/gro) in the ovulatory process," *Methods and Findings in Experimental and Clinical Pharmacology*, 22(10), 725-730 (December 2000).
3. Takahashi, K., Kitao, M., "Effect of TJ-68 (*shakuyaku-kanzo-to*) on polycystic ovarian disease," *International Journal of Fertility & Menopausal Studies*, 39(2), 69-76 (March-April 1994).
4. Mai, A., Horibe, S., Fuseya, S., Iida, K., Takagi, H., Tamaya, T., "Possible evidence that the herbal medicine *shakuyaku-kanzo-to* decreases prostaglandin levels through suppressing arachidonate turnover in endometrium," *Journal of Medicine*, 26(3-4), 163-174 (1995).
5. Ohkura, T., Isse, K., Zkazawa, K., Hamamoto, M., Yaoi, Y., Hagino, N., "Long-term estrogen replacement therapy in female patients with dementia of the Alzheimer type: 7 case reports," *Dementia*, 6(2), 99-107 (March-April 1995).

Eight-Ingredient Pill with Rehmannia

1. Shoji, M., Sato, H., Hirai, Y., Oguni, Y., Sugimoto, C., "Pharmacological effects of *gosha-jinki-gan-ryo* extract, effects on experimental diabetes," *Nippon Yakurigaku Zasshi - Folia Pharmacologica Japonica*, 99(3), 143-152 (March 1992).
2. Kamei, A., Hisada, T., Iwata, S., "The evaluation of therapeutic efficacy of *hachimi-jio-gan* (traditional Chinese medicine) to rat galactosemic cataract," Journal of Ocular Pharmacology, 3(3), 239-248 (Fall 1987).
3. Kamei, A., Hisada, T., Iwata. S., "The evaluation of therapeutic efficacy of *hachimi-jio-gan* (traditional Chinese medicine) to mouse hereditary cataract," *Journal of Ocular Pharmacology*, 4(4), 311-319 (Winter 1988).

4. Sakamoto, S., Kudo, H., Kawasaki, T., Kasahara, N., Okamoto, R., "Effect of *ba-wei-di-huang-wan (hachimi-jio-gan)* on thymidine kinase and its isozyme activities in the prostate glands in rats," *American Journal of Traditional Chinese Medicine*, 16(1-2), 29-36 (1988).

Ephedra Decoction

1. Ozaki, Y., "Studies on antiinflammatory effect of Japanese Oriental medicines (kampo medicines) used to treat inflammatory diseases," *Biological and Pharmaceutical Bulletin*, 18(4), 559-562 (April 1995).
2. Wang, C. M., Ohta, S., Shinoda, M., "Studies of chemical protectors against radiation. XXIX. Protective effects of methanol extracts of various Chinese traditional medicines on skin injury induced by X-irradiation," *Yakugaku Zasshi—Journal of the Pharmaceutical Society of Japan*, 110(3), 218-224 (March 1990).
3. Wang, C. M., Ohta, S., Shinota, M., "Studies on chemical protectors against radiation. XXVII. Survival effects of methanol extracts of various Chinese traditional medicines on radiation injury," *Yakugaku Zasshi—Journal of the Pharmaceutical Society of Japan*, 109(12), 949-953 (December 1989).

Frigid Extremities Formula

1. Xu, F.H., Uebaba, K., "Effect of kampo formulations (traditional Chinese medicine) on circulatory parameters," *Acupunture and Electrotherapy Research*, 24(1), 11-28 (1999).

Ginseng Formula to Nourish the Nutritive Qi

1. Harigai, E., Nakai, S., Kawakita, T., Nomoto, K., "Combined treatment with *ren-shen-yang-rong-tang* (Japanese name: *ninjin-youei-to*) plus prednisolone on adjuvant-induced arthritis in Lewis rat," *International Journal of Immunopharmaoclogy*, 17(50), 411-418 (May 1995).
2 Nakai, S., Kakita, T., Nagasawa, H., Himeno, K., Nomoto, K., "Thymus-dependent effects of a traditional Chinese medicine, *ren-sehn-yang-rong-tang* (Japanese name: *Ninjin-youei-to*),in autoimmune MRI-MP-lpr/lpr mice," *International Journal of Immunopharmacology*, 18(4), 271-279 (April 1996).
3. Kamei, T., Kumano, H., Beppu, K., Iwata, K., Masumura, S., "Response of healthy individuals to ninjin-yoei-to extract—enhancement of natural killer cell activity," *American Journal of Chinese Medicine*, 26(1), 91-95 (1998).

Goddess Formula

1. Huang, K. C. *The Pharmacology of Chinese Herbs* (Boca Raton, Florida: CRC Press, 1993), p. 251.

2. Xue, J. X., Yan, Y. Q., Jiang, Y., "Effects of the combination of *Astragalus membranaceus* (Fisch.) Bge. (AM), *Angelica sinensis* (Oliv.) Diels (TAS), *Cyperus rotundus* L. (CR), *Ligusticum chuangxiong* Hort. (LC) and *Peaonia veitchii* Lynch (PV) on the hemorheological changes in 'blood stagnating' rats," *Chung-Kuo Chung Yao Tsa Chih—China Journal of Chinese Materia Medica*, 19(2), 108-10, 128 (February 1992).

Kudzu Formula

1. Nagasaka, K., Kurokawa, M., Imakita, M., Terasawa, K., Shiraki, K., "Efficacy of *kakkon-to*, a traditional herbal medicine, in herpes simplex virus type 1 infection in mice," *Journal of Medical Virology*, 46(1), 28-34 (May 1995).
2. Ibid.

Ledebouriella Decoction that Sagely Unblocks

1. Bensky, D., Gamble, A., Bensky, L., Kaptchuk, T. *Chinese Herbal Medicine: Materia Medica*, Revised Edition (Seattle: Eastland Press, 1992), p. 33.
2. Yoshida, T., Sakane, N., Wakabayashi, Y., Umekawa, T., Kondo, M., "Thermogenic, anti-obesity effects of *bofu-tsusho-san* in MSG-obese mice," *International Journal of Obesity & Related Metabolic Disorders*, 19(10), 717-722 (October 1995).
3. Morimoto, Y., Sakata, M., Ohno, A., Maegawa, T., Tajima, S., "Effects of *bofutsusho-san*, a traditional Chinese medicine, on body fat accumulation in fructose-loaded rats," *Nippon Yakurigaku Zasshi*, 117(1), 77–86 (January 2001).

Licorice, Wheat, and Jujube Decoction

1. Takahashi, M., Fukunaga, H., Kaneto, H., Fukudome, S., Yoshikawa, M., "Behavioral and pharmacological studies on gluten exorphin A5, a newly isolated bioactive food protein fragment, in mice," *Japanese Journal of Pharmacology*, 84(3), 259–265 (November 2,000).

Major Bupleurum Formula

1. Goto, M., Hayashi, M., Todoroki, T., Seyama, Y., Yamashita, S., "Effects of traditional Chinese medicines (*dai-saiko-to*, *sho-saiko-to*, and *hachimi-zio-to*) on spontaneously diabetic rat (WBN/Kob) with experimentally induced lipid and mineral disorders," *Nippon Yakurigaku Zasshi—Folia Pharmacologica Japonica*, 100(4), 353-358 (October 1992).
2. Shoda, J., Matsuzaki, Y., Tanaka, N., Miyamoto, J., Osuga, T., " The inhibitory effects of *dai-chai-hu-tang* (*dai-saiko-to*) extract on supersaturated bile formation in cholesterol gallstone disease [letter]," American Journal of Gastroenterology, 91(4), 828-830 (April 1996).

3. Saku, K., Hirata, K., Zhang, B., Liu, R., Ying, H., Okura, Y., Yoshinaga, K., Arakawa, K., "Effects of Chinese herbal drugs on serum lipids, lipoproteins and apolipoproteins in mild to moderate essential hypertensive patients," *Journal of Human Hypertension*, 6(5), 393-395 (October 1992).
4. Fushitani, S., Minakuchi, K., Tsuchiya, K., Takasugi, M., Murakami, K., "Studies on attenuation of post-ischemic brain injury by kampo medicines—inhibitory effects of free radical production," *Yakugaku Zasshi—Journal of the Pharmaceutical Society of Japan*, 115(8), 611-617 (August 1995).

Major Construct the Middle Formula

1. Nagano, T., Itoh, H., Takeyama, M., "Effects of *Dai-kenchu-to* on levels of 5-hydroxytryptamine (serotonin) and vasoactive intestinal peptides in human plasma," *Biological Pharmacology Bulletin*, 23(3), 352–353 (March 2000).
2. Murata, P., Hayakawa, T., Satoh, K., Kase, Y., Ishige, A., Sasaki, H., "Effects of *Daikenchu-to*, a herbal medicine, on uterine and intestinal motility," *Phytotherapy Research*, 15(4), 302–306 (June 2001).

Minor Bluegreen Dragon Decoction

1. Yamada, H., Nagai, T., "In vivo antiinfluenza virus activity of Kampo medicine *Sho-seiryu-to* through mucosal immune system," *Methods and Findings in Experimental and Clinical Pharmacology*, 20(3), 185–192 (April 1998).
2. Anonymous, "Japan's Health Ministry Confirms Efficacy of Another of Tsumura's Kampo Drugs," *Kampo Today*, 2 (1), 3 (February 1997).
3. Sakaguchi, M., Iizuka, A., Yuzurihara, M, Ishige, A., Komatsu, Y., Matsumiya, T., Takeda, H., "Pharmacological characteristics of *Sho-seiryu-to*, an antiallergic Kampo medicine without effects on histamine H1 receptors and muscarinic cholinergic system in the brain," *Methods & Findings in Experimental & Clinical Pharmacology*, 18(1), 41-47 (January-February 1996).

Minor Bupleurum Decoction

1. Hirayama, C., Okumura, M., Tanikawa, K., Yano, M., Mizuta, M., Ogawa, N., "A multi-center randomized controlled clinical trial of *Shosaiko-to* in chronic active hepatitis," *Gastroenterologica Japonica*, 24(6), 715–719 (December 1989).
2. Akbar, S.M., Yamamoto, K., Abe, M., Ninomiya, T., Tanimoto, K., Masumoto, T., Michitaka, K., Horiike, N., Onji, M., "Potent synergistic effect of sho-saiko-to, a herbal medicine, during vaccine therapy in a murine model of hepatitis B virus carrier," *European Journal of Clinical Investigation*, 29(9), 786–792 (September 1999).
3. Okita, K., Sakaida, I., Hino, K., "Current strategies for chemoprevention of hepatocellular carcinoma," *Oncology*, 62 Suppl 1, 24–28 (2002).

Polyporus Decoction

1. Sugaya, K., Nishizawa, O., Noto, H., Sato, K., Sato, K., Shimoda, N., Otomo, R., Tsuchida, S., "Effects of Tsumura *chorei-to* and Tsumura *chorei-to-go-shimotsu-to* on patients with urethral syndrome," *Hinyokika Kiyo—Acta Urologica Japonica*, 38 (6), 731-735 (June 1992).

Relax the Channels and Invigorate the Qi Formula

1. Wang, C.M., Ohta, S., Shinoda, M., "Studies on chemical protectors against radiation. XXIX. Protective effects of methanol extracts of various Chinese traditional medicines on skin injury induced by X-irradiation," *Yakugaku Zasshi*, 110(3), 218-224 (March 1990).

Six-Ingredient Pill with Rehmannia

1. Naeser, M. A. *Outline Guide to Chinese Herbal Patent Medicines in Pill Form with Sample Pictures of the Boxes: An Introduction to Chinese Herbal Medicines*, Second Edition (Boston: Boston Chinese Medicine, 1996) p. 292.
2. Yu, S.J., Tseng, J., "*Fu-Ling*, a Chinese herbal drug, modulates cytokine secretion by human peripheral blood monocytes," *International Journal of Immunopharmacology*, 18(1), 37-44 (January 1996).

Stephania and Astragalus Formula

1. Wang, C. M., Ohta, S., Shinota, M., "Studies on chemical protectors against radiation. XXVII. Survival effects of methanol extracts of various Chinese traditional medicines on radiation injury," *Yakugaku Zasshi—Journal of the Pharmaceutical Society of Japan*, 109 (12), 949-953 (December 1989).
2. Zhang, B. Z., Ding, F., Tan, L.W., "Clinical and experimental study on yi-gan-ning granule in treating chronic hepatitis B," Chung-Kuo Chung Hsi i Chieh Ho Tsa Chih, 13(10), 597-599, 580 (October 1993).
3. Zhao, X. Z., "Effects of *Astragalus membranaceus* and *Tripterygium hypoglancum* on natural killer cell activity of peripheral blood mononuclear in systemic lupus erythematosus," *Chung-Kuo Chung Hsi I Chieh Ho Tsa Chih*, 12(11), 669-671, 645 (November 1992).
4. Tang, W., Eisenbrand, G., *Chinese Drugs of Plant Origin: Chemistry, Pharmacology, and Use in Traditional and Modern Medicine* (Berlin: Springer-Verlag, 1992), p. 196.

Tea-Herb Antitode

1. Higaki, S., Kitagawa, T., Kagoura, M., Morohashi, M., Yamagishi, T., "Correlation

between *Propionibacterium acnes* biotypes, lipase activity and rash degree in acne patients," *Journal of Dermatology*, 27(8), 519–522 (December 2000).

Ten-Significant Tonic Decoction

1. Zheng, R.K., "*Shi-quan-da-bu-tang* (Ten Significant Tonic Decoction), SQT. A potent Chinese biological response modifier in cancer immunotherapy, potentiation and detoxification of anticancer drugs," *Methods & Findings in Experimental & Clinical Pharmacology*, 14(9), 725-736 (November 1992).
2. Sugiyama, K., Ueda, H., Ichio, Y., "Protective effect of *juzen-taiho-to* against carboplatin-induced toxic-side effects in mice," *Biological Pharmacology Bulletin*, 18(40, 544-548 (April 1995).
3. Ohnishi, Y., Fujii, H., Hayakawa, Y., Sakukawa, R., Yamaura, T., Sakamoto, T., Tsukada, K., Fjimaki, M., Nunome, S., Komatsu, Y., Saiki, I., "Oral administration of a Kampo (Japanese herbal) medicine *Juzen-taiho-to* inhibits liver metastasis of colon 26-I,5 carcinoma cells," *Japanese Journal of Cancer Research*, 89(2), 206-213 (February 1998).
4. Muraishi, Yo, Mitani, N., Yamaura, T., Fuse, H., Saiki, I., "Effect of itnerferon-alpha A/D in combination with the Japanese and Chinese traditional herbal medicine *juzen-taiho-to* on lung metastasis of murine renal cell carcinoma," *Anticancer Research*, 20(5A), 20931-3947 (September-October 2000).
5. Mori, H., Niwa, K., Zheng, Q., Yamada, Y., Sakata, K., Yoshimi, N., "Cell proliferation in cancer prevention: effects of preventive agents on estrogen-related endometrial carcinogenesis model and on an in vitro model in human colorectal cells," *Mutation Research*, 480-481, 201-207 (1 September 2001).
6. Dai, Y., Kato, M., Takeda, K., Kawamoto, Y., Akhaud, A., Houssain, K., Suzuki, H., Nakashima, I., "T-cell-immunity-based inhibitory effects of orally administered herbal medicine *juzen-taiho-to* on the growth of primarily developed melanocytic tumors in ret-transgenic mice," *Journal of Investigational Dermatology*, 117(3), 694-701 (September 2001).
7. Hidaka, S., Okamoto, Y., Nakajima, K., Suekawa, M., Liu, S.Y., "Preventive effects of traditional Chinese (Kampo) medicines on experimental osteoporosis induced by ovariectomy in rats," *Calcified Tissue International*, 62(3), 239-246 (September 1997).
8. Abe, S., Ishibashi, H., Tansho, S., Hanazawa, R., Komatsu, Y., Yamaguchi, H., "Protective effect of oral administration of several traditional Kampo-medicines on lethal Candida infection in immunosuppressed mice," *Nippon Inshinkin Gakkai Zasshi*, 41(2), 115-119 (2000).

Tonify the Middle and Augment the Qi Formula

1. Yoshida, H., Tanifuji, T., Sakurai, H., Tashiro, H., Ogawa, H., "Clinical effects of Chinese herbal medicine (*hochu-ekki-to*) on infertile men," *Hinyokika Kiyo—Acta Urologica Japonica*, 32 (2), 297-302 (February 1986).

2. Sudo, K., Honda, K., Taki, M., Kanitani, M., Fujii, Y., Aburada, M., Hosoya, E., Kimura, M., Orikasa, S., "Effects of TJ-41 (Tsumura *Hochu-ekki-to*) on spermatogenic disorders in mice under current treatment with adriamycin," *Nippon Yakurigaku Zasshi—Folia Pharmacologica Japonica,* 92(4), 251-61 (October 1988).
3. Cho, J. M., Sato, N., Kikuchi, K., "Prophylactic anti-tumor effect of *Hochu-ekki-to* (TJ41) by enhancing natural killer cell activity," *In Vivo,* 5(4), 389-391 (1991 Jul-Aug).
4. Ikeda, S., Kaneko, M., Kumazawa, Y., Nishimura, C., "Protective activities of a Chinese medicine, *hochu-ekki-to,* to impairment of hematopoietic organs and to microbial infection," *Yakugaku Zasshi—Journal of the Pharmaceutical Society of Japan,* 110(9), 682-687 (September 1990).

True Warrior Decoction

1. Sane, F., Komatsu, Y., Amagaya, S., Chisaki, K., Hayashi, H., "Effects of 9 Kampo medicines clinically used in hypertension on hemodynamic changes induced by theophylline in rat," *Biological Pharmacology Bulletin,* 23(6), 762–765 (June 2000).

Uncaria Formula

1. Mimaki, Y., Toshimizu, N., Yamada, K., Sashida, Y., "Anti-convulsion effects of choto-san and chotoko (Uncariae Uncis cum Ramlus) in mice, and identification of the active principles," Yakugaku Zasshi, 117(12), 1011-1021 (December 1997).
2. Goto, H., Yang, Q., Kita, T., Hikiami, H., Shimada, Y., Terasawa, K., "Effects of Choto-san on microcirculation, serum nitric oxide and lipid peroxides in patients with asymptomatic cerebral infarction," *American Journal of Chinese Medicine,* 29(1), 83–89 (2001).

White Tiger Formula

1. Nakashima, N., Kimura, I., Kimura, M., Matsuura, H., "Isolation of pseudoprototimosaponin AIII from rhizomes of *Anemarrhena asphodeloides* and its hypoglycemic activity in streptozotocin-induced diabetic mice," *Journal of Natural Products,* 56(3),345-50 (March 1993).

Index